EBM Guide For Scientists to Sales Reps

Medical Evidence in the World of Payers & Health Care Systems

A Handbook For Industry to Better Understand, Communicate and Navigate These Worlds

Delfini Group Evidence-based Practice Series

By Sheri Ann Strite and Michael E. Stuart MD

"Best help with evidence-based medicine available."
Marty Gabica, MD, Chief Medical Officer, *Healthwise*

First Edition: 02/2014
ver: 20140221
Delfini Group Publishing: Delfini Group LLC
http://www.delfinigrouppublishing.com

ISBN-13: 978-1496041210 (CreateSpace-Assigned)
ISBN-10: 1496041216

Cover Design: Sheri Ann Strite
Cover Photo Credit: NASA/JPL
Bridge Photo Credit: Sheri Ann Strite

With much gratitude to our reviewers and advisors in these three worlds, with special thanks to DM, GN, HK, JC & MM.

Table of Contents

Disclaimer

Use of this information implies agreement to our Notices at— www.delfini.org/index_Notices.htm.

In addition, your use implies agreement to the following. **We make no warranty, express or implied, or representation as to the accuracy, sufficiency or continued currency of the information contained herein.** The information contained in this book and any information or documents from the Delfini website may not be appropriate for use in all circumstances. Information may not be up-to-date, and it is up to the user to update the information.

WHY YOU WANT TO READ THIS BOOK: BRIDGE BUILDING

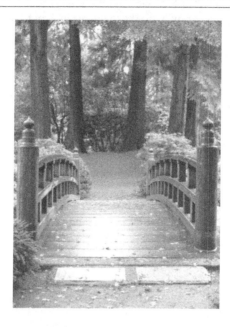

If men can be said to be from Mars and women from Venus, then it is at least as fair to say that those working in health care systems or companies that provide coverage for health care and those working in the drug and medical technology manufacturing industries often relate to each other as if they come from different planets—which, indeed, they do. We've written this book to **help those working in industry bridge these planets and foster a good relationship with both health care systems and payers using medical research to help establish meaningful common ground and a common language, with the ultimate goal of best serving patients.**

We come from the payer- *and* health care systems-planet, but on the provider side. Typically, in our world, physicians and pharmacists who leave to work in industry are jokingly (or not so jokingly) said to have gone over to the "dark side." Imagine our surprise then, when teaching a group of industry scientists, analysts and account directors, one of them told us that for a while he left pharma to go work on the dark side. "Which would be *where*?" we asked in puzzlement, thinking we had misheard. All the workshop attendees started laughing at our confusion. "Well, on the *payer* side, of course," he answered, laughing himself.

And so we have a situation in which key players who have a major impact on health care decision-making, and ultimately on health outcomes, view each other in drastically opposing—and not very complimentary—terms. This can't be good for patients. And worse, much of the opposition—and confusion—centers on medical research, which we will interchangeably refer to as evidence or medical science, and which is where, as medical information scientists, evidologists and clinical improvement experts, we spend much of our lives.

The overarching mission of this book is to better serve patients. And patients will be best served when everyone engaged in their care is focused on their benefit: this includes manufacturers, providers of care and payers of that care. To help advance our mission of serving patients, our goal for this book is to help those working in industry better understand medical decision-making and the use (and sometimes misuse or nonuse) of scientific evidence by payer and health care systems to support or reject the coverage or benefit determination of a therapeutic intervention.

Unless they are unified under one company (and sometimes, even when they are), health care systems and payers are very different entities—but when it comes to medical evidence, there are big similarities. Each necessarily has to be cognizant of a population view and many of these organizations have their own pharmacy and therapeutics (P&T) and medical technology assessment (MTA) committees. For purposes of this book, the information we provide here is useful in working with each group. For simplicity's sake, frequently we will just use the term "customer" to refer to payers or health care systems unless we have something unique to say about one or the other. And while the focus of this book is on the microcosms of the health care systems and payer worlds, much of the information here, including tips, may be relevant at times to any medical decision-maker, including the prescribing physician or any other health care professional engaged in some way in medical decision-making.

To achieve our goal, our objectives for this book are to help bridge the world of manufacturers and the world of payer and health systems customers by helping industry to—

1. Better understand health care systems, payers and other customers with a focus on their varying approaches to medical research;

2. Be aware of typical confusions and misunderstandings by customers about medical science;

3. Be attuned to typical research design, performance and reporting gaps that may hurt acceptance of your products—and what you can do to remedy this;

4. Develop greater common ground and a common language to employ with customers in discussions about the medical evidence; and,

5. Effectively harness the power of medical evidence to connect and communicate with customers.

This book is about helping you navigate the world of your customers whether they are sophisticated about medical research or not.

This book is written for anyone and *everyone* working in industry who is involved in—

- Generating or communicating about research; and,

- Any one of you who may face a research comment or question coming from a customer or who may be instrumental in facilitating such a discussion.

That means that this book is written for scientists as well as those in contracting or sales and everyone else in between such as product teams, scientific liaison staff, medical communications staff, etc. We will explain **why this book is useful for those of you who generate and report on research,** but let us **start first with those of you who directly interact with customers.** Many of you think of "communicating about the science" as being the responsibility of scientists and medical science liaisons. But the more you know about some essential basics about discerning the quality and clinical usefulness of research may help you better do your job. For example, consider this—

To Those In First-line Communications With Customers: A Scenario for You

The more you understand about an evidence-based approach, the more skilled you will be at working with your customers, and you may become the pivotal point for a yes or no coverage decision or a decision to keep your product's placement on a drug or technology formulary.

An evidence-based approach employs critical appraisal which, for our purposes, means evaluating medical research for its likely **reliability** and its **clinical usefulness.** Importantly, **understanding basic elements of critical**

appraisal is not hard, and you can understand a lot about study results by simply understanding **a few easy-to-understand statistics** which utilize **extremely simple** mathematical formulas. The point of this book is not to teach you critical appraisal (and you do not need that knowledge for this book to be useful to you); but an objective of this book is, in part, to encourage you to gain basic critical appraisal knowledge. We are known for our simplified approach to understanding critical appraisal concepts, and we will give you choices of resources to help you.

The more you understand about critical appraisal, the more skilled you will be at determining the critical appraisal ability of your customers, understanding their evidence-based philosophy and evaluating what they are, or are not, putting into practice. This will potentially increase the success of your discussions with customers, which can make a crucial difference in a review or contracting decision.

Let us start by imagining a scenario in which you are representing a new drug on the market that high quality studies have shown to be highly efficacious and for which only a few minor side effects have been reported. The new product, however, is priced higher than the longstanding alternative. You are talking to a pharmacy director, and he tells you that his team has just completed a review of your new agent and various alternatives. He challenges you. Why, he asks, should they use your drug when the number-needed-to-treat reported in your competitor's studies is smaller? Their agent will help more people, according to their research, yet your agent costs more.

This might be a make-or-break moment for your company. Your hope is that he will let you arrange for an appointment with your scientific team. But merely offering a meeting with your team could—at best—delay a change in perception about your agent and—at worst—could close the door, resulting in "end-of-discussion."

Your best option is to give the director a response that keeps the door open for discussion. And how do you do that? Because he has issued you a critical appraisal challenge, the best option is to answer him using a critical appraisal response.

Number-needed-to-treat—or NNT—means the number of people that need to be treated within a certain period of time for one patient to experience a benefit over the compared alternative. On the surface, the lower the number, the better. However, if you have a sufficient understanding of critical appraisal, you know that there can be many reasons why an NNT could be smaller *other* than your competitor's product being more effective than your agent. Knowing this, you have a greater chance to address what may be an incorrect conclusion on the part of the pharmacy director. You also increase chances for further engagement and a changed position on your agent.

Your response could go something like this:

"I'm sure you know there are a lot of reasons why the number-needed-to-treat could be 'reported' as being smaller, but the actual truth of effect could be very different.

- I'm sure you know that bias tends to favor the intervention being studied which can make a reported NNT falsely small.

- It could be explained by heterogeneity in the studies such as a difference in study populations, study methods or in patient experiences or other differences.

- It could be a chance effect.

- Depending upon how it was derived, there could be issues with calculation methods.

"There are ways to look closely at all these areas, and I would be happy to arrange for one of our medical science liaisons to meet with you to discuss the studies you've reviewed and look into it more deeply."

Or you might be in a situation in which your customer knows relatively little about what constitutes a high quality study. If the science behind your product is strong and the science behind your competitor's product is poor, you have an opportunity. For example, care may have been taken to conceal patient assignment to their study groups in your study and no such measures were taken in your competitor's studies. You might say, "Research has shown that weaknesses in studies can falsely inflate results—sometimes even making results appear to be favorable when, in fact, they aren't. I would be happy to bring someone in to talk about our science and explain very transparently how our methods protect our studies from bias. For example, for blinding to be successful, it's important to make sure that no one is able to know or affect which study group a patient gets assigned to. I would be very happy to bring in one of our scientific staff members to talk with you about this."

Frequently, you get only one shot. In this book, we will give you some tips for how you can use some basic understandings about these types of customers and about medical evidence to help keep the door open. The more you understand about critical appraisal of the medical literature—regardless of your specific role—the greater an asset you are to your company.

This is true whether you directly communicate anything you learn about critical appraisal or just listen with a knowing ear. You may be the reason that a decision turns in your company's favor when good evidence and good reporting support the superior value of your products.

While this book is **not** intended to teach you critical appraisal, we will address selected critical appraisal concepts as they pertain to general problems with study quality and reporting or typical misunderstandings on the part of many customers.

And, importantly, even if this is very new to you, don't worry! Again, the good news is that it is not difficult to acquire a basic understanding of the general elements needed for critical appraisal. Much of the time, a general understanding of bias and chance may be sufficient to evaluate whether or not an interventional research study is likely to be reliable and clinically useful. Frequently, the key to understanding the reliability of a study is not about statistics, but is about study design, methodology, execution and study performance outcomes such as whether or not blinding was successful. Armed with basic critical appraisal knowledge, you may understand your customer better, you can participate in discussions more flexibly and helpfully, you may hear something important to pass along to others on your team, and potentially you may do a world of good.

To Those Generating and Reporting Medical Research

Why will this book be helpful to you? You may be among the best researchers in the world, and yet much in this book has been written to benefit you.

Many of you think of the Food and Drug Administration (FDA) as your customer, neglecting to view payers or health care systems as your customers too. If you count yourself among these kinds of scientists, you may be missing some important opportunities that may help patients and, worse, your good work may be rejected due to misunderstandings by these customers or because key information that they need is not available to them.

We have worked with many industry scientists who are shocked when they learn how many of their studies might fail a critical appraisal and be rejected by customers. Frequently scientists are insulated from these end-users and, as such, are often not aware of what users are looking for to help them in their medical decision-making. In this book, we describe in detail elements for successful reporting, and we also discuss design elements and study methods that are frequently cited as being of import to customers.

We also provide you with "evidence about the evidence" to support our claims and observations about what we consider to be an unfortunate medical misinformation mess that you can be instrumental in helping to solve.

Also, many of you will become involved in directly communicating about your science to customers at some point. We help you understand some typical pitfalls and some common misunderstandings they may have, and we will give you helpful tips to navigate the world of these customers which differs in many ways from your own.

To All

An important truth to keep in mind as you read this book is that **we are all rooting for reliable and useful science**. A chief problem is that *many of your customers don't know how to tell what that is.* Another chief problem is that *many of you aren't providing the right information for those who do.*

BEFORE WE GET STARTED, A FEW CONVENTIONS & NOTES

We have organized this book in **two parts** which are equally important. The first part of this book is conversational in style to provide you with general information. In some instances, we have greater elaborations or details to share with you which we have placed in **appendices** to serve as the second part of this book and which can be found *after* **About the Authors**. The appendices too are conversational in style, but take a deeper dive into details for selected sections.

You will find that we repeat information and concepts at times. This is generally because we want individual sections to be sufficiently complete without you having to search out related information.

References

References are generally labeled as [author name and publication year]. The citation can be looked up in the alphabetized reference list at the end of the book. The PubMed Identification (PMID) numbers in the citations can be entered into the PubMed search box at http://www.pubmed.gov to access the study abstract.

Resources

We will provide you with access information to a **Reader Resource** web page at the end of this book where you can find additional resources including an online **glossary**. In addition, a wealth of **freely available** and helpful resources can also be found at our website: www.delfini.org. The **Reader Resource** web page also includes **hyperlinks** to most of the URLs listed here.

Medical Research Study Types

Unless otherwise specified, we will only address **medical research of therapies and involving human subjects.**

Critical Appraisal

Critical appraisal is a core activity of evidence-based medicine (EBM) and, in this context, refers to the evaluation of medical research for its likely **reliability** and its **clinical usefulness.** For research of medical therapies, we are interested in whether associations between an intervention and an outcome are due to cause and effect—or whether study **bias**, such as lack of blinding, or **chance** explain or distort results. In the context of a study, bias means something other than chance that leads away from truth. **"Research or study quality"** is a shorthand way of alluding to the likely reliability of research results.

To determine whether study results are likely to be reliable, we evaluate the study for **validity**, or closeness to truth. There are two large validity categories. **"Internal validity"** is the term for understanding how true the study is in its own context. **"External validity"** addresses how true the results are likely to be in medical practice. When we say **"validity,"** we will be referring to internal validity. In speaking of external validity, we will always label it as such.

We will **interchangeably use the terms** "critical appraiser," "reviewer," "evaluator," "appraiser," etc., to mean anyone—payers, health care systems and others such as ourselves—who perform an evaluation of a study for reliability and clinical usefulness. Note, however, that when we talk about "critical appraisal," we are **strictly referring to the action of someone performing an appraisal—not whether they have performed an appraisal well.** A key point of this book is that **there is great variability** in the quality of critical appraisals, which we will also refer to at times as "reviews" or "evaluations," etc. **A key question for you is whether it is likely or not that a reviewer has performed an adequate critical appraisal.** We will provide you some tips for trying to gauge this.

This book is about helping you navigate the world of your customers whether they are doing critical appraisals or not—and whether they are doing *high quality* critical appraisals or not.

We will explain a number of critical appraisal concepts—and you may learn a lot about critical appraisal by reading this book. However, again because the purpose of this book is **not to train you in critical appraisal, this book is not intended to be complete on that topic.** For those of you who wish to go beyond this book, the book listed below, others that we recommend at our website at www.delfini.org or other resources that you can find on your own that covers similar material, will be of use to you:

> **BASICS FOR EVALUATING MEDICAL RESEARCH STUDIES:**
> **A Simplified Approach**
> **And Why Your Patients Need You To Know This**
>
> **Delfini Group Evidence-based Practice Series**
> **Short How-to Guide Book**

We will, however, include as **APPENDIX F the** *Delfini Short Critical Appraisal Checklist—Interventions For Prevention, Screening & Therapy.* This checklist should be considered to be **in shorthand** and so it is not explanatory. However, it will give you a one-place itemization of the essential core concepts of critical appraisal for these types of studies.

General Notes

- We are **generalizing**, and there are **exceptions** to everything we say.

- We are aware that there are **constraints on industry communications with customers, but we will be ignoring these**. Things change, companies interpret things differently, etc. Therefore, for the purposes of this book, we are going to advise you as if no constraints exist. We can provide you with our best help if we leave it to you and your company to determine how you can apply what we share with you.

- And, lastly, often the best general critical appraisal answer to just about anything is, "It depends." The reason for this answer is that a "threat" to the validity of a study may or may not bias the results depending upon other details of the study.

WHEN IT COMES TO MEDICAL EVIDENCE, THIS IS THE ENVIRONMENT OF HEALTH CARE SYSTEMS & THIS IS THE ENVIRONMENT OF THE PAYER

So let us talk about the health care system or payer customer and their world as it relates to medical decision-making and medical evidence. As stated, one of our objectives is to help you better understand these kinds of customers—and most particularly with an eye on medical evidence. Increasingly, payers and health care systems are including some form of an evidence-based evaluation in their reviews of drugs, biologics, devices and other interventions. However, there is great variation in the ability of your customers to discern evidence quality, and there are some typical misunderstandings and confusions many of your customers have about specific study elements.

There is also great variation in the quality of the available evidence and its reporting. As we have stated, another important aim of ours is to describe some study design and performance issues and the gap we often see between scientific conduct and what gets reported in a scientific paper. Missed opportunities in scientific reporting are often the reasons for the rejection of many otherwise high quality research studies. Customers who do understand how to critically appraise a study might not take the time and trouble to seek out missing information and may label your study as of "uncertain risk of bias," passing it by in favor of studies with the information they seek in a scientific paper.

Therefore, in this section we want to toggle between the **world of customers, the world of medical manufacturing and the world of medical evidence.** Our discussion will center around these topics—

1. Why FDA approval is frequently not sufficient for customer acceptance of a product;

2. Satellite view of evidence quality issues;

3. Industry and customer perceptions of each other;

4. Customer variation in approaches to evidence; and,

5. Evidence and customer medical decision-making.

THE PAYER, HEALTH CARE SYSTEMS AND THE FDA

When It Comes to the Science, The FDA Is Not Your Only Customer (Though Some of You or Your Colleagues Think That It Is)

We have a long history of working with industry. We also have a long history of working with health care systems and payers—including the fact that we, ourselves, worked for many years in an integrated delivery network. And so it came as a surprise to us when we began doing some programs a few years ago, aimed at helping industry better understand what customers and others need by way of science and scientific reporting, that we came to learn that many in industry only think of their science as something directed toward the FDA. *If the FDA accepts their research*, the thinking went, *everyone else will.*

But this is not true. Evidence-savvy customers do not approve drugs or devices just because they have FDA approval. Instead many do their own critical appraisals to assess study quality and clinical usefulness—and they should. We will discuss why this is. And so importantly—

FDA Point #1: FDA approval is not a guarantee of customer acceptance of a product. If you do not view your health care system and payer customers as equally important as the FDA as a "customer of your science," you may miss important opportunities with these customers and may even find that your product is rejected.

Trust and the FDA: When It Comes to the Science, FDA Involvement Is *Not* A Guarantee of Study Quality and Clinical Usefulness

Many industry scientists at those industry-facing programs we held were generally unaware and surprised that we and others evaluate the quality of the medical science ourselves and that doing so requires disclosure of very specific information in the publication or in other accessible resources. The prevailing sentiment that we heard from industry scientists and others was that everyone should at least accept, without question, any science that was conducted or supported by industry if it was a trial conducted for regulatory approval *because* of the very close involvement by the FDA.

Study quality can be compromised by study bias or risk of chance effects. The fact of the matter is that there is great variation in the quality of research *even* when the FDA is involved. While the FDA often does very good work, skills in the area of understanding what constitutes high quality medical science vary—and this is true throughout the health care world. FDA staff come from the same pool as other medical decision-making professionals, and effective training in understanding what constitutes quality in medical science is frequently lacking in medical and pharmacy schools and elsewhere.

Therefore, some pivotal trials are of low quality, FDA medical reviews vary in quality, and decisions at times contradict recommendations from advisors. Lastly, there may be varying reasons for FDA approval that are independent of study quality.

We will give you greater insights into study quality generally, but the bottom line is—

FDA Point #2: FDA involvement in your research is *not* a guarantee of a high quality clinical trial.

Also, be aware that, just because the FDA wants a particular outcome, does not mean that *that* outcome is of particular interest to a customer. In fact, customers not infrequently express frustration with selected outcomes that may have been chosen by the FDA (and often without their being aware of FDA involvement, laying any criticisms squarely and unfairly at the feet of the manufacturer). For example, the FDA used to accept hemoglobin A1c as an acceptable outcome without other clinically meaningful outcomes, such as cardiovascular events, which are desired by end-users. And even if an outcome in your trial is important, other outcomes important to customers may be missed.

FDA Point #3: Outcomes desired by customers may be missing in your studies.

Which leads us to—

Trust and the FDA: Even When There Are High Quality, Clinically Useful Studies, FDA Approval is Not Enough

So when we and others *are* in agreement with the FDA over study quality and outcomes, why might a customer not settle for FDA's acceptance without conducting their own review? There are several reasons why reliance upon the FDA is insufficient for medical decision-makers' sole source of information about the efficacy and safety of drugs and devices.

For one thing, a customer may be interested in a specific question not being asked by the FDA. Questions can differ, and questions drive a review: For example, the question, "Do the benefits of this therapy outweigh the risks?" may result in a very different kind of review than the question, "How does this therapy improve treatment, safety and value for patients with a given disease compared to other treatment options?"

The agency does not provide any information about comparative efficacy and safety or cost or compare options in other ways. (And "comparative effectiveness research" or CER will not necessarily be *the* answer, which we address in **Appendix B**: *"Real World Data."*) Usually health care systems and payers are interested in interventions in the "context" of other available alternatives. This context can be very complex, involving a myriad of considerations often beyond efficacy and safety—issues we refer to in shorthand as "triangulation issues" such as cost, patient perspectives, clinician satisfaction, employer considerations, public relations, risk management, etc. We will provide a detailed list of such considerations in the section, *MEDICAL DECISION-MAKING & THE COMMITTEE*.

Also, there are many instances in which reviewers may disagree that there is *sufficient* evidence of efficacy and safety. A single clinical trial—even if assessed to be at low risk of bias—may—

1. In fact, be highly subject to study bias in ways undetectable in the available information about the study;

2. Report results that are chance effects;

3. Be selectively reported, omitting some important information that could change the picture; or,

4. Be fraudulent.

Therefore, we are made much more comfortable about the efficacy outcomes of assumably valid studies when more than one study has been done by groups with differing interests in slightly different ways (so as to avoid replication of study biases resulting from copying another's design) and reporting similar results.

Safety is another matter entirely. Most clinical trials are constructed to answer efficacy questions. Safety issues are less likely to be discovered in efficacy studies as adverse events are relatively rare, and initial studies are frequently small and of short duration. Findings of no statistically significant difference in safety outcomes may be reflective only of an insufficient number of people studied to uncover a meaningful difference and/or too short trial duration. Sometimes the collection of safety information is not as rigorous as the collection of data to support the study's aim, and sometimes the reporting of safety data in trials is poor.

FDA Point #4: The bottom line is that satisfying the FDA does not necessarily result in satisfying the needs of others who are customers of your science as well.

Having given you some background to help you understand potential customer reactions and responses to FDA decisions, let us now move more deeply into the world of evidence and the customer. To do so, you first need some greater background into the world of scientific evidence quality for medical interventions generally—and what we have to say may really surprise you.

MEDICAL EVIDENCE & THE EVIDENCE AND THE CUSTOMER: IN BROAD STROKES

As strange as this may sound, the appropriate use of science in medicine is actually fairly new. Understanding about what is required for study reliability continues to be something that is studied and evolves. Plus understanding what constitutes scientific quality has not been successfully integrated into the training of most health care professionals who will be engaged in medical decision-making, and it is from this base that many scientists come, along with editors, peer reviewers, clinicians, academicians, etc. And so, we have a situation in which customers vary wildly in how they relate to medical evidence, which is one of the key points of this book. Industry professionals need to understand basic critical appraisal concepts to most effectively deal with this wide variation.

This book will provide you with more detailed insights into what is required for scientific quality. And again, if this is new to you, don't worry because we will explain things in simple terms, and the concepts we describe should be relatively easy to understand. For now, what we want to impress upon you is that we and other groups with a good knowledge of what constitutes quality in medical science have estimated that **much of the medical literature is of uncertain reliability or is not reliable**—this is true *even* in journals considered to be of the highest quality. Further, much research conducted for the purpose of examining what constitutes study quality—what we refer to as "the evidence-on-the-evidence"—has demonstrated that bias in studies tends to favor the intervention of interest under study. This means that frequently bias makes study outcomes look better than they actually are—and potentially even favorable when they are not. Let us go into this a little more deeply.

The Health Care Information Problem: A Lot of Research and A Lot of Potentially Untrustable Research

It will come as a surprise to many of you that we have a large problem with the quality of information we get from the published medical literature. This is regardless not only of FDA involvement and journal reputation, as we have mentioned, but also irrespective of the reputation of research centers and scientists.

1. In discussions concerning the state of scientific knowledge, the Institute of Medicine (IOM) concluded that it was plausible that only 4% of interventions used in health care have strong evidence to support them [Field 92].

2. And yet, we have a lot of studies. The National Library of Medicine (NLM) is the world's largest library. At this writing, PubMed comprises over 22 million citations for biomedical literature, and each week more than 13,000 references are added to it [PubMed FAQ].

3. Professor John Ioannidis "...charges that as much as 90% of the published medical information that doctors rely on is flawed [Freedman 10]."

4. It is our estimate, having evaluated thousands of studies, that less than 10% of published randomized controlled trials (RCTs) in the health care literature are both valid and clinically useful or reported sufficiently to tell.

5. One large review of 60,352 studies reported that only 7% passed criteria of high quality methods and clinical relevancy [McKibbon 04].

6. Fewer than 5% passed a validity screening for a highly respected evidence-based journal [Glasziou 06].

7. One study concluded that there may be considerable bias in p-values reported in abstracts [Gotzsche 06].

8. Much of the time, the chief problems with medical research reliability are due to bias. Bias in studies tends to favor the intervention. Bias has been documented to distort results up to a relative 50% or more for many individual biases. [Chalmers 83, COTS 07, Juni 01, Juni 99, Kjaergard 01, Lachin 00, Moher 98, Nuesch 09, Poolman 07, Schulz 95, Shih 02, Tierney 04, van Tulder 09]

9. One study found that 18 to 68% of abstracts in 6 top-tier medical journals contained information not verifiable in the body of the article [Pitkin 99].

10. We've talked about problems with understanding safety. The bottom line is that safety information is usually quite limited, and months or years may pass before we truly know about safety—if ever.

Evidence Point #1: The vast majority of published medical science articles are not reliable or clinically useful or are of uncertain reliability.

The Health Care Information Problem: What's Wrong?

What's wrong is that there is an enormous lack of understanding of what constitutes good medical research by most professional medical decision-makers such as physicians and clinical pharmacists. This means that many interventional decisions made are not supported by high quality science. It is vitally important that you understand the magnitude of this problem.

Typical study flaws include—

1. Lack of balance or uncertainty of balance in prognostic variables between patient groups for study (shorthand "unequal" or "unbalanced groups"). The term "prognostic variables" refers to demographic and clinical factors (e.g., age, blood pressure, etc.) that are known or believed to influence a subject's likelihood of responding or reacting to an intervention. Having similar groups is important because, to isolate a cause and effect relationship, everything in a study must be identical between study groups except for what is under study;

2. Inappropriate comparators;

3. Lack of blinding;

4. An imbalance between groups in co-interventions or care experiences— again, important because everything must be identical except for the intervention being studied. (Example: In a study comparing a medical treatment to a surgical treatment, bias is likely if the surgical patients receive more frequent visits than the medical group because they may feel better because of getting extra support or there might be more known about their outcomes because of this extra attention.);

5. Insufficient treatment or follow-up duration;

6. Problems with measurement methods;

7. Meaningful missing data;

8. Lack of transparency in analysis methods or analysis choices which favor the intervention under study; and,

9.   Problematic reporting of results.

There are many other types of study flaws, but this is just to give you a flavor of some of the most common problems that can result in an assessment that a study is at high risk of bias.

The widespread lack of critical appraisal skills results in the publishing of many flawed studies reporting beneficial results which, in fact, are inflated or erroneous. This can affect you in numerous ways. Let's take a scenario in which your research is of high quality, but your competitor's is not. They might report results that appear, at first glance, to be more favorable, but the real reason for more impressive results is bias which has inflated their results. Your best position is always to understand the key critical appraisal outcomes for your company's studies and those of your competitors—this is true whether you directly communicate information about evidence to customers or not. Armed with this information, you may learn something of import from your customer that you would not have otherwise known is meaningful and which you can pass along knowledgably to others with whom you work with less likelihood of your mistranslating the problem.

When we say that there is a widespread lack of critical appraisal skills, the problem is even bigger than you might think. It certainly surprised us when we first started doing this work. You might find illuminating the questions and results of our critical appraisal pretest.

Question 1.

You read a report that 240 patients presenting with a number of symptoms are treated with Nuevo-Magico—a drug used for many years in Europe for various indications, and just approved by the FDA in the US. Symptoms are sometimes severe enough that people are confined to bed for a period of days. People may be ill for weeks. The disease is highly contagious and can be dangerous in the elderly. The side effects of Nuevo-Magico are documented in numerous well-done studies to be very rare—less than 1% have an allergic reaction, usually presenting as a mild rash. No long-term adverse effects have been reported over many years. Of the 240 patients treated, 232 patients are asymptomatic within 3-5 days of coming into the doctor's office. Because of a special program, there is no cost to patients.

Would this convince you that this agent would be appropriate for patients similar to those tested? If yes, why? If no, why not?

Remarks:

Nearly 80% of physicians and 90% of clinical pharmacists tested **failed** this question because they did not notice the absence of a comparison group. (In fact, at the last place that we taught this, upon the "reveal," a physician cried out with some embarrassment, "Oh, no! And I suppose this is something self-limiting like a cold or the flu!" That is exactly right.)

Question 2.

Before we get to the question, here's a quick primer in case this is helpful to you. An **absolute difference** between groups is obtained by simple subtraction between the percentage of outcomes in each group. Example: if 15% of patients in the control group experience a heart attack and 10% of patients in the intervention group experience one, the **absolute risk reduction** (ARR) is 15 minus 10 for an ARR of 5%. Whereas, a **relative measure** is a proportion. Ten is proportionally smaller than 15 by one third, and so the relative risk reduction (RRR) in our example is 33%. And so the reduction can be described as a 5% reduction or a 33% reduction, even though these numbers are expressing differences for the exact same outcome. (*Which sounds better to you—and everybody else?*) Relative measures cannot be smaller than absolute measures. They can be equal, but that is very rare. Almost always they are larger—and frequently much larger.

Here's the question—

A well done study reports a statistically significant relative risk reduction of 60% for patients in the intervention group, with a modest side effect profile. Would this convince you that this agent would be appropriate for patients similar to those tested? If yes, why? If no, why not?

Remarks:

Over 70% of physicians we tested leaped to yes—and, therefore, **failed**. Clinical pharmacists fared better at a failure rate of nearly 60%. It was this reported "amount of benefit" that helped Vioxx become a blockbuster drug when the absolute benefit was less than 1%—and which, as most of you know, did *not* have a modest side effect profile. So the relative risk reduction for clinically important upper gastrointestinal events was 60% of less than 1%, thereby benefiting only one out of 125 patients in comparison to naproxen.

It is shocking how many physicians and clinical pharmacists have not been taught the difference between absolute and relative measures—especially when you consider how easy it is to calculate the absolute difference and how important it is to know it as compared to the relative measures.

Question 3.

A study reports that 4.4% of 1629 patients are unavailable for their Intention-To-Treat analysis. No data were imputed. Comments?

Remarks:

Failure rates for this question are high as many people have never heard of intention–to–treat analysis, and those who have heard of it frequently misunderstand it. Intention–to–treat analysis requires that some value be obtained or—if missing—assigned for all patients randomized in the study and that patients be analyzed in the groups to which they are randomized. For dichotomous variables (meaning one of two choices, such as alive or dead), intention–to–treat analysis has been recommended to be the primary analysis method for efficacy outcomes of superiority trials by editors of major journals. And yet, it is seldom performed, is seldom performed correctly or is frequently biased in the choice of imputation method. And end-users rarely know they need to evaluate it or understand how to do so.

We have trained thousands of people in the methods of critically appraising medical research. We've trained people in school, immediately out of school and seasoned professionals. We've trained different *kinds* of professionals—physicians, clinical pharmacists, faculty, residents and students, nurses, quality improvement leaders and even judges and consumers. We have trained people in different kinds of groups—government, payer, health care system, medical writers, content development, etc.—and we've trained people from all around the country. We've worked with schools and at schools. We frequently see the following pattern: schools in the United States are, for the most part, not effectively teaching students of the health care professions how to appropriately evaluate validity and clinical usefulness of medical research—let alone interpret it—and that's because many faculty doing the teaching are unskilled in this area and unaware.

Evidence Point #2: The health care information problem is primarily one of insufficient training. In part, this often results in poor quality research or research of uncertain quality. Further, many health care decision-makers lack skills to differentiate high quality and useful research from that which is of low or uncertain quality and/or clinical relevance—and, what's more, many don't even know that they need to.

Further, their ability to understand research results is often flawed or lacking.

The Health Care Information Problem and the Experts

So the experts can help us out of this mess—*right?* Systematic reviewers and meta-analysts surely understand how to evaluate clinical trials for quality and clinical usefulness, providing us with a summary of reliable evidence. We must have a wealth of reliable help from professional society clinical practice guideline teams that are filled with experts. Whole businesses are dedicated to creating other guidance for us such as compendia and other secondary sources of medical information. At the national level, vast resources have been made available for CER (comparative effectiveness research). We have a wide array of talent involved in constructing complicated economic models to assess cost-effectiveness of various interventions. Can't we just rely on these?

Alas, the answer is no. We have personal experience with all of these sources and know directly of many, many problems. And we are not alone.

Systematic reviews, of which a meta-analysis is a subtype, can be complex to do and, unfortunately, often researchers include low quality studies: "The inclusion or exclusion of trials of low methodologic quality has a substantial impact on results and conclusions from systematic reviews and meta-analyses" [Egger 03]. Many meta-analyses are exploratory in nature and include small trials, thereby increasing risk of small-trial bias. Further, when well-done RCTs are conducted after hypothesis-generating meta-analyses, the results often do not confirm the initial results of the meta-analysis [Brok 08, Hennekens 12-09; Hennekens 04-09]. "The outcomes of the 12 large RCTs we studied were not predicted accurately 35% of the time by the meta-analyses published previously on the same topics" [Le Lorier 97].

In one review of 431 clinical practice guidelines produced by US medical specialty societies, 82% did not apply explicit criteria to grade evidence, 87% did not report whether a systematic search of the literature was performed, and 67% did not describe the type of professionals involved in the development of the guideline [Grilli 00]. One study reported that almost half of the guidelines appearing in journals such as the Annals of Internal Medicine, BMJ, JAMA, NEJM, Lancet and Pediatrics do not cite RCTs [Giannakakis 02].

And then there are compendia. A drug compendium is a summary of important drug information for selected agents. Compendia are used by some customers (e.g., Medicare) to make coverage and reimbursement determinations for pharmaceutical products. However, we and many other users do not rely on drug compendia because of concerns about the quality of information. In one review of drug compendia, the Agency for Healthcare Research and Quality (AHRQ) found that only a small proportion of the available evidence was considered, and the included trials were frequently of low quality [AHRC 09].

Pharmacoeconomic analyses combine several elements into an economic model in an attempt to predict what may happen in clinical practice. The elements that create the model include health care outcomes, which should be based on valid and useful randomized controlled trials, cost data and assumptions such as the estimated number of patients who will be prescribed a particular medication and the number of patients who will experience various outcomes including adverse events. However, most pharmacoeconomic studies are of low quality because of undue emphasis on cost (a local consideration) without assessing the quality of the evidence regarding efficacy and safety [Jefferson 02, Stone 05].

We could go on and on...

Evidence Point #3: The health care information problem extends to nearly all sources of information. "Experts" come from the same pool as others working in this area and frequently lack sufficient training in critical appraisal. Secondary studies such as meta-analyses and secondary sources such as clinical guidelines, compendia and cost-effectiveness studies are frequently rife with medical science that is not reliable and/or is not clinically useful.

The Health Care Information Problem and the Customer

It should now come as no surprise to many of you that the vast majority of customers are part of this large group of health care decision-makers who 1) lack awareness of the health care information problem; and, 2) lack skills to be able to differentiate high quality and useful research from that which is of low quality or uncertain quality and/or lacking in clinical relevance.

As one insightful industry colleague, Michael Donabedian, pointed out to me, "Industry personnel tend to work with what is right in front of them today." Well, what is in front of you today are potential opportunities of which you may be unaware. Having knowledge of essential critical appraisal principles can help you work not only with customers who are performing critical appraisal, but also with those who are not or who lack these skills (or who lack awareness that they need to be doing this work). While not wishing to imply that we think of medical decision-making as a game (we do not), the term "game-changing" has resonance.

And so we wish to emphasize that anywhere within this range of customer know-how and application or lack thereof, is the potential for a game-changing opportunity where good science and its reporting have a chance to face-off with poor quality science or that which is of uncertain quality through gaps in reporting. And what if your competitor understands basic critical appraisal concepts, user needs for reporting, typical gaps in quality and reporting and knows the strengths and weaknesses of research supporting your and your competitors' product?

Furthermore, things are changing. Mike, this same industry colleague said to us, "I think your book needs to be read by every single employee within industry who touches someone managing a population in a health system or a payer or regardless of where or how. Perhaps communicate something to the effect of 'get ready for change, because it is already here... and there is still more to come.' I think this would help industry people realize that they need to be out in front of this, and they need to start educating and preparing today. Your book will help industry both deal with what's going on today regardless of a customer's skills in EBM or use of evidence and help us get way out in front of new practices surrounding health technology assessments."

Okay, so we are saying it, "*Get ready for change, because it is here!*"

But a key point is that even if it were not—**even if not a single customer of yours knew anything about evaluating the quality of medical science**—your understanding critical appraisal principles can help you be more effective at your job.

However, awareness of the health care information problem and what to do about it will only increase over time. As we have stated, increasingly customers are including some form of an evidence-based evaluation in their reviews of drugs, biologics and other interventions. And even among those who are not, we see a greater sense of uncertainty and even, at times, a discomfort that something is not right in the medical science universe. We all see headlines, such as "Why Most Published Research Findings are False," by the renown clinical epidemiologist, John Ioannidis [Ioannidis 05], "Unreliable Research: Trouble at the Lab" [The Economist 13] and "FDA official: 'clinical trial system is broken'" in the BMJ [Cohen 13]. Oh, yes, and twenty years ago there was the BMJ editorial, "The scandal of poor medical research," [Altman 94] and then the twenty year update to that in the BMJ, "Medical research—still a scandal," [Smith 14]. These articles provide a tiny biopsy of the myriad problems in medical science—and even customers who aren't evidence-mavens are increasingly uncomfortable with the reliability and relevance of medical science. We used to experience more surprise and shock when, during teaching sessions, we enumerated typical problems in medical science. Now, more often, we get, "I'm not surprised."

Customer & Evidence Point #1: Most customers lack skills in evaluating study quality, but awareness of the need to assess study quality is growing. However, even if it were not—even if not one single customer of yours knew anything about evaluating the quality of medical science— your understanding critical appraisal principles is a strength.

Customer Perceptions of Industry & Evidence

Some of this lack of surprise has to do with the fact that so much of published medical science is funded or conducted by industry, and it will come as no surprise to anyone reading this that there is discomfort with industry and with industry involvement or support in research. Consequently, a typical question that we get during our critical appraisal training programs from clinicians is whether or not they should simply avoid all research that is conducted or supported by industry.

Our response to that question is a resounding, *no.* If they did that, they would miss important studies that can provide them with information that is important to patients. We also point out that *everyone* involved in research should be assumed to be biased.

An academic scientist with no industry ties should be expected to be interested in the benefits of positive research results. Researchers generally choose to study something because they believe it works. That scientist will likely have put in considerable time and investment into his or her work and, understandably, desires to have that work result in a meaningful outcome. That scientist is likely to want recognition and its resulting benefits, as would most anyone else. That scientist may well be in a "publish or perish" situation in his or her academic department or may need to get published in order to secure tenure. There is, of course, a certain amount of fraud that happens in research. We suspect that this is more likely where there is less oversight. And for this reason, FDA involvement in some industry research may help mitigate fraud that might be more likely to happen without their involvement. The bottom line is that *all researchers* should be assumed to be potentially biased and should be assumed to be biased in favor of what it is that they are studying.

Based upon what we have shown you about the evidence-on-the-evidence, we and other evidence-savvy reviewers put the greatest trust in science that has high quality reporting and can stand up to a rigorous critical appraisal regardless of the funder or industry involvement. We make *note* of industry involvement; however, only with rare exception does industry involvement figure into our conclusions about the reliability and usefulness of a study.

Customer & Evidence Point #2: Most customers are uncomfortable with industry involvement in research, but *all* researchers should be assumed to be biased in favor of what they are studying, irrespective of funding source or affiliation. Quality in studies helps mitigate researcher bias, and transparency in reporting facilitates assessing study quality. But many customers do not understand this.

Industry Misperceptions of Payers & Evidence

Stepping away from health care systems for a few minutes, having spent a lot of our work life in the payer universe for so long, sometimes, when working with industry, we've had flashes of finding ourselves in Bizarro World. As many of you probably know, Bizarro World was a comic creation of the universe *opposite* to that of Superman's (the *Dark Side* versus the *Dark Side,* anyone?). According to Wikipedia, in popular culture... "'Bizarro World' has come to mean a situation or setting which is weirdly inverted or opposite of expectations."

And this is the way we are using it—to mean *opposite*—and not necessarily bizarre. But we like the term, because it highlights how extreme at times the variances in thinking can be, further illuminating that frequently we are on different planets.

Our first experience of a Bizarro moment happened when we were attending a presentation for both payers and industry in which a brilliant and talented evidence-savvy clinical pharmacist presented his critical appraisal of a clinical trial. We were both very impressed with his analysis and his presentation of it. We felt that he did a great job of describing how he approached his review and in detailing his documentation of the many biases and other study problems that he had identified.

Following his presentation, Sheri exclaimed to a couple of industry colleagues of hers, "That presentation was incredible!"

Her colleagues completely shocked her when they exclaimed, "It was! It shows us how payers will go to *any* lengths to reject a study!"

Not only is this type of thinking wrong, this kind of thinking will not help you in working with payers and other medical decision-makers. It simply widens the chasm between groups and deepens an adversarial stance—which is not in the best interest of patients. Most payers and health care system customers are not required to take an evidence-based approach. It is expensive and time-consuming to do so, and usually the only reason for a payer or health care system to perform a systematic review and critically appraise evidence is because they actually understand that the quality of science matters for quality patient care and reducing waste.

We want to move you away from typical industry thinking that we've heard that goes roughly like this—

- "They are doing critical appraisal to reject studies!"

- "What evidence do you have that it *doesn't* work?"

- "The FDA was very involved—this was a pivotal trial. What authority do you have to question this study?"

To thinking more like this—

- "They are doing critical appraisal because they are concerned about the reliability of the science. Without reliable evidence, predictions about what will happen (benefits and harms) by choosing various interventions may be wrong. Doing critical appraisal is important for the quality of patient care."

- "I need to supply you with convincing evidence that our intervention works."

- "Despite involvement of the FDA, I understand that you, as a consumer of our science, need to be able to evaluate its quality and clinical usefulness for yourself because of your role as a steward of the quality of care for patients and as a steward of resources."

Customer & Evidence Point #3: Generally, customers that invest in evidence reviews—whether the reviews are of high quality or not—are doing so because they are trying to be responsible and do the right thing for patients.

"The Ugly Baby Syndrome" versus "We *Want* to *See* the Baby!"

Our industry-facing programs helped us to see that there is an especially huge chasm between industry and payers. This chasm is characterized by some serious misperceptions which this book hopes to address. Following the initiation of our programs, we started hearing rumors of hurt feelings resulting from the stated needs to evaluate the quality of the science. As one scientist said to us in an injured tone, "You're saying that my *baby* is *ugly!*"

Again, the foreignness of the notion that we and others need to evaluate the science ourselves was pressed upon us practically physically. As physicians go—or anyone, for that matter—Mike is a very approachable guy. He is very friendly and is in no way intimidating, partly because he is such a nice guy, but also because he is rather short in stature. At this program, hands over their hearts, tall and imposing scientists would loom over Mike and loudly proclaim in some distress, "I've been *doing* science for *over 30 years!*" To which, Mike would look up, hand-over-heart right back at them, and proclaim, "And I've been *reading* science for *over 30 years!*"

Things came to a head when we were hired by a company to do some staff training and, at the start of our workshop, one of the scientists challenged us, saying something to the effect of, "Even if we have not reported the specifics of randomization, for example, you should assume that we have done this and have done this correctly! We are among the best scientists in the world!"

"I believe that you are," Mike countered. "However, the evidence does *not* support that we should trust the reported results of studies if key methodological considerations are not sufficiently described in the publication. We don't even need to see much description often. But we do need some kind of statement that computer-generated randomization was used, for example."

He then proceeded to put up a slide of results from a Cochrane Collaboration study which supported his claim. The Cochrane Collaboration is a well-respected worldwide group of more than 31,000 volunteers that conducts systematic reviews of randomized controlled trials of health care interventions. Keep in mind that research has shown us that bias tends to inflate reported results, generally favoring the intervention under study. In this particular review of studies, low quality studies reported almost twice the amount of benefit as high quality studies. In studies in which study procedures and other study elements were unclear, they also reported nearly twice the benefit as reported in higher quality studies—suggesting that studies of uncertain quality were as biased as the low quality studies [Hartling 09].

When presented with this information, our scientist colleague nodded in surprised agreement and expressed that he was now convinced that complete and clear reporting was more important than he had thought. So, in fact, if your company has done high quality research, show it off because we *want* to see it. **We *want to* see *the baby!*** (For those of you who are interested in the specifics of this

Cochrane study, the outcomes are described in greater detail in **Appendix E** along with greater details about the evidence-on-the-evidence and potential impacts of bias on study results.)

Customer & Evidence Point #4: We all want high quality research. Customers that invest in evidence reviews are looking for high quality research. To determine if research is high quality, transparency in reporting is required.

Which leads us to...

Cost and Waste and Value

We all know that money is a prominent issue in health care. We all know that both medical and pharmacy costs are increasing at huge rates. Regardless of who writes our paycheck, this affects us all. Payers, for certain, have to pay attention to this regardless of their business model or their profit status. (Clinicians *should* pay attention to this, but frequently do not—often to the detriment of patients—and health systems may vary, again, depending upon their business model.) Cost is not the focus of this book, but we do want to point out that financial considerations include cost, value and waste.

When it comes to cost, there are some health care systems and some payer groups—and probably even some clinicians—that couch financial decisions as being based on evidence when they are not. We think this does a disservice to everyone. Science should not be forced into servitude to a decision that is actually financially- or otherwise-based. We tell people, "Go ahead and make a decision on any basis that you want. But do not call it an evidence-based decision when it is not." We point out that an expensive intervention may, at some point, not be expensive. If they are not upfront about the reasons for their decisions, they may have put themselves—and potentially patients—in situation that will be awkward at best and possibly even untenable at its worst due to precedent setting.

That said, waste is directly related to medical science quality. Waste occurs when the resources required for an intervention are not commensurate with the value of the resulting outcomes. We were once hired by a drug company to develop a clinical practice guideline for irritable bowel syndrome for which they had a recently approved agent. The company was startled when our first recommendation in the guideline was for dietary change despite *any* high quality science to support its likelihood of benefit—which we stated right in the guideline.

"We thought you were the *evidence experts!*" they exclaimed. We then explained that an evidence-based approach does not necessarily exclude interventions that are not supported by the evidence. Among other things, an evidence-based approach requires that you identify relevant research and evaluate it. It also requires transparency. Our process and resulting output met both of these requirements. Also, in this particular case, there was also no evidence suggesting that dietary change would not work. The dietary changes that we were recommending would not result in harms or many additional costs to patients. The drug, however, was expensive, and its use carried the risk of side effects—known and unknown. Therefore, prioritizing dietary change as a first step, despite a noted lack of support of the evidence, was reasonable, responsible and fit with the value equation.

Value can only be determined after information about the quality and usefulness of science is known. An evidence- and *value*-based approach to quality improvement requires a systematic review and synthesis of the evidence regarding benefits, harms or risks, but also costs, alternatives and uncertainties of health care interventions as well as an assessment of the trade-offs between effectiveness, cost, the patient's perspective and the organization's priorities, etc., meaning other triangulation issues [Strite 05].

In our training programs, we encourage people to focus first on the quality of the medical science and its potential usefulness to patients. When at Group Health, Mike—who had chaired the P&T committee—was asked to take responsibility for medical technology assessment. Prior to Mike's involvement, we had a massively dysfunctional committee. Mike's response was to recommend that the committee be reconfigured into two committees. He would take responsibility for the first committee whose entire focus was on the quality and usefulness of the science. As Mike puts it, that committee would then "throw the evidence over the wall" to the second committee made up of medical directors, which would then be responsible for decision-making. That second committee would have the evidence from Mike's committee and could then focus on a variety of decision-making considerations such as cost, legal ramifications, consumer preference, etc. We don't think that it is a necessary requirement for best evidentiary practice to have a separate group to evaluate the evidence and a separate group for decision-making. But what we do think is that it is necessary to *first* focus cleanly and clearly on the science without regard to other considerations which will affect coverage decisions.

Customer & Evidence Point #5: Many customers have to pay close attention to waste and value. Evidence-savvy customers know that careful review of the evidence can aid in this effort.

When You've Seen One Payer, You've Seen One Payer; When You've Seen One Health Care System, You've Seen One Health Care System

While payers do share some commonalities such as a need to pay attention to cost, waste and value, there are some interesting differences. Despite the commonality of holding the purse strings for many medical interventions, how attention to cost plays out may vary depending upon the obligations and business model of the company or payer entity such as how it is governed, legal considerations, community perspectives and pressures, etc.—in short, many of the triangulation issues. So too is there great variation with different health care systems that is dependent upon a whole host of factors.

For example, during the time that we worked at Group Health Cooperative in Seattle, "Group Health as a payer" was less prominently positioned by leadership than "Group Health as a health care system." As all payers are, we were very concerned about cost. As a not-for-profit health care system, we had limited funds, we needed to use them wisely for the benefit of our consumers and so attention to cost was vitally important. However, we were also a *consumer-owned* health care cooperative, and, as such, the members were primarily focused on the quality of their care—that was the reason for our very existence. We both worked in the clinical improvement division where our mantra was, "If we focus on quality, cost may follow." Sometimes the use of quality evidence resulted in health care initiatives that cost us a lot, but we engaged in them anyway because we believed it was the right thing for patients. More frequently, however, we believed that effective use of science was steering us away from waste and frequently, from potential patient harms.

Government, as a payer too, has to pay close attention to cost, but is also required to take a perspective that includes a quality focus as a caretaker of special populations and as a steward of tax payer dollars.

Contrast these with other kinds of payer organizations, such as for-profits, whose outlook may also be very cost-centric, but motivated differently, especially where their directives are to maximize their profits and which potentially could be at the expense of patients' best health care options.

The point is that cost matters—but how that plays out may vary radically, resulting in differing coverage or tiering decisions (which, from here on out, we will generally just refer to as "coverage decisions").

Payers, health care systems and other customers who are evidence-sophisticated, however, are more likely to operate from greater common ground. We want to stress "more likely" and not necessarily the same. There are many reasons why even more skilled evidence-reviewers may have differing takes on the same evidence and may differ in their critical appraisals such as—

1. Critical appraisal is frequently an act of discovery and comprises knowledge of critical appraisal concepts, clinical knowledge and critical thinking. Different reviewers will differ in discoveries made and in knowledge, skills and aptitude.

2. Reviewers may be very skilled, etc., but be very pressed for time which may limit their ability to do the research and analysis needed for a thorough review—especially if needed information is absent from the publication.

3. Differing clinical questions may result in different reviews for the same product.

4. Critical appraisal is very context-specific to the individual study, but some customers choose to standardize critical appraisal approaches for consistency or to save time.

5. Judgment is required—and different individuals may make different judgments.

That said, people who do a good job at critical appraisal will frequently agree about the likely reliability of a study and are generally open to information that helps them do an effective appraisal. And while judgment is a necessary component of critical appraisal, an evidence-centric approach by a skilled appraiser tends to be a neutralizer.

Customer & Evidence Point #6: Payers and many health plan customers have to pay close attention to cost, waste and value, but how they do so may vary, depending upon many factors. Evidence-savvy customers may be less likely to vary because quality evidence, at times, serves more as an equalizer.

Two Kinds of Customers

One of the big differences between customers is how they relate to evidence. So at a really crude level, we actually can say that there are two kinds of customers: those who look primarily at cost and those who look at study reliability before looking at results and *then* look at cost and other considerations "in light of" the evidence. As we have described, in this latter group there is a great deal of variation in knowledge and skills. However, this latter group of customers is growing and gaining in numbers.

What this means to you is that whomever you are dealing with on the customer side (and this may be multiple people) could be all over the map when it comes to understanding medical science. It is important to keep in mind that critical appraisal is often a journey of discovery and that decision-making may be very fluid as other considerations are evaluated. The more you know about critical appraisal, the more effective you may be in communicating with medical decision-makers.

A medical science liaison, for example, is well-advised to understand about bias and why study results can be hugely magnified by biases in a given study. Judgment is required in rating the risk of the various biases, and useful conversations with customers can occur when discussants are all knowledgeable about bias, confounding (a special form of bias) and the play of chance. In such situations, healthy "give and take" and valuable learning can occur during conversations.

For example, many evidence discussions will include considerations around what we refer to as "grey-zone" evidence. The grey zone refers to evidence that is of borderline reliability or usefulness, and different assessors may reach different conclusions about the benefits and risks of these studies. Industry professionals knowledgeable about critical appraisal may contribute important information to evidence discussions (e.g., by educating customers about weighting various biases) which may help a customer recognize when evidence is in fact borderline—not inconclusive—and this may make it more likely that a customer will accept a new intervention which may have value to a patient.

A key part of this book is going to be to give you some tips to help you figure out where the person you are communicating with is on the evidence-based knowledge continuum. To do this successfully means that you are going to need to have a working exposure to critical appraisal principles. The more you can understand of these principles, the more effective you will be at your job—with the bonus outcome that you will have the potential to be a more informed patient and helpmate to your loved ones and friends.

Customer & Evidence Point #7: It is important to understand the evidence sophistication of the customer organization you are working with, how they evaluate the evidence and the evidence sophistication of the individuals in the organization who are involved in the review of your product. The more you understand about critical appraisal of the

medical literature, the more you will be able to assess this and the better you will be able to communicate both with evidence-savvy customers and those who are not.

The Train Has Left The Station—The Question Is *Who* Is Driving The Train And *Where* Is It Going?

When it comes to evidence, there are customers at two ends of a continuum—

1. There are customers who understand what it means to have valid and clinically useful evidence—and who know how to assess validity and clinical usefulness and do so.

2. There are those who have little such understanding.

3. Importantly, there is a wide spectrum in between.

4. In addition, there can be some complex scenarios that present different challenges to navigate.

5. There are customers who have staff who have critical appraisal skills, but who do not provide the resources—mainly in the way of time or enough skilled people—to do the work.

6. And there are those who say they are evidence-based, but in reality are not. The term "evidence-based" is frequently merely a buzz word.

Some groups simply rely upon the FDA or will be likely to accept any randomized controlled trial just because it is an RCT. But that group is shrinking.

Some staff within some customer organizations have very strong critical appraisal skills, and some organizations support critical appraisal work. But many have minimal to modest skills or may know key critical appraisal concepts, but they may become rigid in their application of the concepts. A rigid approach may occur when skills are not robust or because of other factors such as lack of time to conduct thorough appraisals or seek out additional information such as information that was not supplied in the publication.

Having said all of this, over time we have seen an increasing *interest* in better understanding the evidence and increasing *interest* in how to evaluate it. (This doesn't necessarily mean that these medical decision-makers are better equipped to understand *how* to evaluate and apply evidence, but it does mean that evidence is becoming more of a focal point.) This could be a good thing for patients if people have clarity about what it truly means to have an evidence-based approach. But in fact, this sometimes results in a bit of a confusion. All the more reason for you to understand what is required for high-quality science and clinical usefulness. Your role then can broaden not only to be an advocate for your products, but also an educator.

The following quote well expresses what we are increasingly hearing over time:

> "I am a Managed-Care based Clinical Pharmacist with a strong desire to sharpen my skills in critical appraisal. There is so much misinformation in the literature these days. Cost becomes an issue when comparing two or more equally safe and efficacious agents. The challenge is arriving at the determination of the safety and efficacy part…not to mention [whether the agent is] clinically useful. I am certainly not convinced that just because a drug has FDA approval all is well in the world. In the best interest of our patients, the physicians deserve an unbiased, evidence-based recommendation from me regarding drug reviews. Trustworthy medical literature is lacking. I want to make recommendations that can be clinically justified. I am concerned that we tend to let our guards down just because an article was published in JAMA or BMJ. Someone once said, 'We all see only that which we are trained to see.' "

Customers are doing things differently than in the past, and this is evolving. Customers and others are looking at evidence differently, and momentum is growing. What does this mean for industry? We believe that this means that those companies who choose to become fully engaged in evidence discussions with customers will be increasingly seen as true partners and will gain credibility and trust.

We have seen this in action. When companies have chosen to engage us for teaching evidence-based principles, we have seen a marked increase in collegiality toward account managers and those responsible for organizing those programs because of value and transparency. We have watched doors open. When companies have done a good job of transparently and completely reporting the evidence for high-quality studies, we've seen coverage decisions change from rejection or uncertainty to acceptance.

Customer & Evidence Point #8: Attention to the evidence and an evidence-based approach is increasing. Industry members who are knowledgeable about a truly evidence-based approach, conversant in evidence-principles and who bring value through an evidence-based approach to customers may be received with greater trust and openness.

MEDICAL DECISION-MAKING & THE COMMITTEE

The actual decision-making, of course, is generally the responsibility of the P&T or MTA committee. The customer may make recommendations—and frequently they do—and clinical guidelines and other sources may be consulted—and frequently are—but usually the deciders are the committee members. The committee staffers may have painstakingly evaluated the evidence, they may have made many other kinds of assessments, they may have carefully outlined what they and others recommend and why. Now the evidence and everything else they've done gets thrown over the wall to the decision-makers. Welcome to the wild and wooly world of the committee where anything can happen—and frequently does.

There are many reasons for decisions about whether drugs and other interventions are placed or maintained on a preferred list or not, how they are tiered and whether they are subject to prior authorization or other conditions on their use, etc. To give you a flavor of these reasons and also to give you a framework for how decision-making might be structured, we present a framework below. **Keep in mind as you review the framework that this is just one example,** and other possibilities are many.

A Framework for Medical Coverage Decision-Making: A Sampling of Decision Considerations

There is the evidence, and then there are "other considerations" which we refer to as the triangulation issues. Here is our list:

- Science: reliability and clinical usefulness of the intervention;

- Patient perspective: benefits, harms, risks, costs, uncertainties, alternatives, applicability, satisfaction, clinical considerations (e.g., tolerability, ease of use, dependency or abuse potential), unmet needs and special populations;

- Clinician perspective including satisfaction; and,

- Other decision considerations: accreditation issues, community standards, cost, customer considerations, ethical considerations, liability and risk management issues, marketing, media or press issues, medical community impacts, medical-legal, public relations, purchasing issues, regulatory, research realities (e.g., no studies providing reliable evidence are likely to be conducted, etc.), utilization and capacity issues, overall impact on the health care organization and other.

End-users will vary in how they approach product coverage decision-making. Below is a simple model of how a hypothetical group might make a coverage decision:

I. Validity: rate the validity of the study evidence (or the body of evidence)—

- The evidence is sufficient to conclude efficacy;

- The evidence is borderline (i.e., the evidence is suggestive, but further studies are needed to clarify); or,

- The evidence is inconclusive.

II. Rate the new product in the light of evidence and existing alternatives in terms of—

- Benefits and risks, patient preferences, utilization, capacity, liability, cost, regulatory, patient preference, and legal issues or other triangulation issues. (Even if the evidence is inconclusive, there may be some instances where important other considerations result in a committee deciding to include a new product.)

When You've Seen One Person, You've Seen One Person

The point is that the committee is made up of individuals—and on committees they tend to behave very—*well*— *individually*. What you thought was going to happen, through what may have been long, tortuous and excruciatingly detailed discussions with customer staff, might ultimately result in a decision that makes you do a double-take and has you pounding the side of your head in complete mystification. (And has your boss calling you, saying, "*What!?!?*")

What happened? Well, maybe what happened is the committee. P&T and MTA committees, even in the most structured groups and even in the most evidence-based groups, are dynamic, and they are often made up of people with strong opinions and who are used to making decisions as individual agents. There are formal leaders, such as committee chairs, but informal leaders emerge in the unique context of the membership present at any particular meeting. Some of these informal leaders are always seen by other members as leaders, although even when this is true, it doesn't mean it is true for every discussion. Sometimes an individual not typically seen as a leader will emerge as one during a review of a specific product. This may happen because of that individual's specialty or his or her stated experience with a product or indication or subpopulation. The experience may be based on a broad range of experience or may be a one-time occurrence that may or may not be factually related to the product. But frequently, in lieu of others having experience in these areas, beliefs about that experience with a therapy or product will frequently drive the outcome.

Product Decision-making Point #1: Regardless of what you experience in your customer-to-industry discussions, the ultimate decision-making milieu may be akin to hanging out on the frontier of the Wild West. Decisions are frequently person-powered. Shots can come ringing out of nowhere, can ricochet, might be duds—anything is possible. What happens depends upon who shows up for the meeting—and part of what happens, and its predictability, depends upon whether those who show up have some understanding of the need for a truly evidence-based approach and if there is someone present who can help make that happen.

People love to have opinions, right? Often substantiated or not. Imagine a typical party-setting—*since we are hanging out on the dark side, Star Wars bar, anyone?* The mood and attitude all depend upon who shows up. People have opinions all over the map and frequently love to express them. Different people emerge as discussion-bearers, assert their opinions or become those deferred to for a host of reasons—sometimes simply because of politesse. So it is in most any committee. And when it comes to P&T and MTA committees, so it especially is with the doctors...

"There is Good Evidence That..."

Let's look a little more closely at some crucially important committee dynamics, using P&T committees as an example, with points relevant to technology assessment committees as well. Typical P&T committee membership is composed, by and large, of physicians and pharmacists. While many pharmacists are active participants of P&T committees, it is the physician membership that generally drives discussions and decision-making—or, in the case of pharmacist participants, their perceptions of the experiences, wishes and needs of the physicians they represent. And we have already shared with you that the likelihood that committee physicians have had much, if any, meaningful exposure to critical appraisal concepts is low.

Many years ago, one of our first big surprises in working with P&T committees occurred when we had spent many months training staffers of a large health plan in evidence-based activities such as critical appraisal and evidence synthesis, working to correct and refine their evidence templates, auditing their work and helping them develop and structure their presentations. We were then invited to attend a first P&T committee meeting following all of this activity. We were so proud of the staffers, who were doing ace reviews and now had very well organized and transparent materials along with succinct presentations that hit all the right points.

It is very common for clinicians to know of some evidence, but really have no idea how to evaluate whether the evidence is reliable or not. Yet frequently physicians are very fond of saying, "*There is good evidence that...*," when there is nothing of the sort—frequently there is weak evidence or, in reality, often they are really just expressing an opinion.

At the first utterance of these words in the P&T committee meeting we observed, the presenting staffer immediately looked down, closed up and slid away. We were shocked. Upon witnessing this repeatedly during this meeting, we came to realize that customers that do not find a way to override the pharmacist's natural deference to a physician and that do not find a way to foster a climate of attention to critically appraised evidence are often wasting any evidence-review efforts.

Here are some scenarios for the interplay between customer staff and medical decision-making committee members—

1. The customer's committee staffing team is not evidence-savvy. The committee is not evidence-savvy. The decision outcomes depend upon a variety of factors such as business model (and even governmental payers can be thought of as having a "business model"), company perspective, leadership positions, the power and opinions of other influential individuals, etc. Without attention to evidence quality, most studies are deemed to be of similar quality. Depending upon the decision drivers, outcomes can be all-comers, no-comers, it's all about cost, it's all about physician preference, etc. It's a collection of judgments with the outcome dependent upon those seen as leaders or who are best at group process (or sometimes, the loudest). This is most common.

2. The customer team is evidence-savvy. The committee is evidence-savvy. In all likelihood this has come about because the customer team has spent time and resources helping the committee reach evidence sophistication. While the decision outcomes depend upon a variety of factors such as those described above, attention is paid to evidence quality. Evidence becomes a neutralizing force in committee discussions. Evidence is generally given great weight in decision-making. Opinions are generally restricted to non-evidentiary items. Decisions may be based on judgment, but—depending upon the business model—most decisions are based on the evidence. This is rare, but increasing.

3. The customer team is not evidence-savvy. The committee is evidence-savvy. In reality, this is not very likely. The closest we have seen this is when there is an individual committee member or two who are evidence-sophisticated. But without needed support work performed by the customer team, decision-making is not likely to be very evidence-based.

4. The customer team is evidence-savvy, but the committee is not evidence-savvy and pays little attention to the work of the customer team who do little to assert themselves in the decision-making discussions of the committee. This is much more common than scenario 2—and look out, because anything can happen.

5. The customer team is evidence-savvy, but the committee is not evidence-savvy. However, the committee makes decisions with close attention to the customer team. When this happens, often this is a result of the customer team taking some proactive steps that foster an evidence approach even when committee members personally lack critical appraisal skills. This may include an effective orientation with members, careful selection of committee leadership, highly transparent review materials, effective evidence-based presentations, just-in-time teaching of key critical appraisal points and their import and, importantly, active participation by the customer team in review discussions.

Product Decision-making Point #2: Physicians on the committee typically drive the decisions; however, if evidence-based practice is allowed to flourish, decision-making is likely to be based on the quality and usefulness of the evidence, decisions may be more predictable and objective, and decisions may be less person-powered and judgment-oriented.

It's All Relative

One way in which we see industry feel perplexed and sometimes overwhelmed by customer decision-making is when they neglect to keep clear about the fact that, in the world of the customer, decisions are typically **comparative**. You may have the best science in the world and even the best treatment for a particular indication, but an alternative option may also have sufficiently good evidence, have a good benefit-to-safety ratio—even if not as good—and be cheaper, thus being perceived as resulting in better value.

Assuming that you are a typical shopper, view the customer through the same kind of lens as you would when you make purchasing decisions. This viewpoint should be taken at the outset all the way through to committee decision-making. Ideally, you want to know how they are viewing your product and its research and whether that review is likely to be fair and balanced. And you want to know what other interventions they are evaluating and how these alternatives compare, with particular attention to how decision considerations may be weighted. And this should be assumed to be unique to such factors as indication, populations, availability of alternatives, etc.

It's All Relative—Except When It Isn't!

And then when it comes to drugs, there is "class effect." Class effect refers to a concept that certain drugs share sufficient similarities that they can be thought of as a class. It is a determination that a set of agents with similar chemical structures, mechanisms of action and pharmacological effects has similar therapeutic and adverse effects. There are no universally accepted criteria for defining class effect. (For all intents and purposes, class effect treats the agents as if they are the same clinically, but some other factors, such as cost, may vary.)

And so while it is true that customers are generally making comparisons, often they may operate using class effect thinking and lump groups of drugs together to do their comparisons. This may result in further Wild Westism when it comes to product decision-making. P&T committees, for example, frequently conduct reviews of a class of drugs because it is a convenient way to organize reviews. However, some committees make the mistake of believing that all agents in a class are interchangeable for various conditions and in various populations. For example, all-cause mortality, acute myocardial infarction and stroke outcomes may differ markedly with the use of various ACE inhibitors (angiotensin-converting enzyme inhibitors) [Furberg 03]. Similarly traditional nonsteroidal anti-inflammatory drugs (NSAIDs) are commonly considered as a drug class. Again, these agents may vary significantly in efficacy and adverse events (e.g., gastrointestinal adverse events) [Ong 2007].

If you have a good product and good science behind it with meaningful clinical outcomes, it is to your benefit to educate customers on the pitfalls of class effect thinking so that your agent gets a fair chance of review and a fair chance to benefit patients.

Frequently, physicians on committees make their decisions based on specific agents, but a customer taking a class effect viewpoint may mitigate that, and decision-making may take on a more lumped-together approach.

Product Decision-making Point #3: Formulary decisions are usually comparative—at least in a broad sense. However, many groups utilize a class effect approach. This is irrespective of evidence-sophistication. We,

however, believe that class effect may not be in the best interest of patients and can be particularly problematic when high quality science with meaningful clinical outcomes becomes obscured or misappropriated because of this approach.

WHEN IT COMES TO MEDICAL EVIDENCE, THIS IS THE ENVIRONMENT OF THE HEALTH SYSTEM AND PAYER CUSTOMER: IN SUMMARY

Let's review the key points of what we have just covered in this section. At the highest level—

I. FDA approval is insufficient for customer acceptance of a product.

II. We have a significant health care information problem composed of concerns about medical science quality and clinical usefulness, coupled with lack of effective knowledge about this problem and skills to deal with it.

III. However, awareness of this problem is growing among customers, and a truly evidence-based approach can help determine a product's value.

IV. Even when your customers lack an evidence-based understanding and/or approach, your knowledge of evidence-based principles can be very important.

V. Decision-making in the context of a committee can be very complex; however, a committee that utilizes a truly evidence-based approach is more likely to make decisions that are more objective and less prone to the judgment of an individual or a few.

Details—

1. FDA Point #1: FDA approval is not a guarantee of customer acceptance of a product. If you do not view your health care system and payer customers as equally important as the FDA as a "customer of your science," you may miss important opportunities with these customers and may even find that your product is rejected.

2. FDA Point #2: FDA involvement in your research is *not* a guarantee of a high quality clinical trial.

3. FDA Point #3: Outcomes desired by customers may be missing in your studies.

4. FDA Point #4: The bottom line is that satisfying the FDA does not necessarily result in satisfying the needs of others who are customers of your science as well.

5. Evidence Point #1: The vast majority of published medical science articles are not reliable or clinically useful or are of uncertain reliability.

6. Evidence Point #2: The health care information problem is primarily one of insufficient training. In part, this often results in poor quality research or research of uncertain quality. Further, many health care decision-makers lack skills to differentiate high quality and useful research from that which is of low or uncertain quality and/or clinical relevance—and, what's more, many don't even know that they need to. Further, their ability to understand research results is often flawed or lacking.

7. Evidence Point #3: The health care information problem extends to nearly all sources of information. "Experts" come from the same pool as others working in this area and frequently lack sufficient training in critical appraisal. Secondary studies such as meta-analyses and secondary sources such as clinical guidelines, compendia and cost-effectiveness studies are frequently rife with medical science that is not reliable and/or is not clinically useful.

8. Customer & Evidence Point #1: Most customers lack skills in evaluating study quality, but awareness of the need to assess study quality is growing. However, even if it were not—even if not one single customer of yours knew anything about evaluating the quality of medical science— your understanding critical appraisal principles is a strength.

9. Customer & Evidence Point #2: Most customers are uncomfortable with industry involvement in research, but all researchers should be assumed to be biased in favor of what they are studying, irrespective of funding source or affiliation. Quality in studies helps mitigate researcher bias, and transparency in reporting facilitates assessing study quality. But many customers do not understand this.

10. Customer & Evidence Point #3: Generally, customers that invest in evidence reviews—whether the reviews are of high quality or not—are doing so because they are trying to be responsible and do the right thing for patients.

11. Customer & Evidence Point #4: We all want high quality research. Customers that invest in evidence reviews are looking for high quality research. To determine if research is high quality, transparency in reporting is required.

12. Customer & Evidence Point #5: Many customers have to pay close attention to waste and value. Evidence-savvy customers know that careful review of the evidence can aid in this effort.

13. Customer & Evidence Point #6: Payers and many health plan customers have to pay close attention to cost, waste and value, but how they do so may vary, depending upon many factors. Evidence-savvy customers may be less likely to vary because quality evidence, at times, serves more as an equalizer.

14. Customer & Evidence Point #7: It is important to understand the evidence sophistication of the customer organization you are working with, how they evaluate the evidence and the evidence sophistication of the individuals in the organization who are involved in the review of your product. The more you understand about critical appraisal of the medical literature, the more you will be able to assess this and the better you will be able to communicate both with evidence-savvy customers and those who are not.

15. Customer & Evidence Point #8: Attention to the evidence and an evidence-based approach is increasing. Industry members who are knowledgeable about a truly evidence-based approach, conversant in evidence-principles and who bring value through an evidence-based approach to customers may be received with greater trust and openness.

16. Product Decision-making Point #1: Regardless of what you experience in your customer-to-industry discussions, the ultimate decision-making milieu may be akin to hanging out on the frontier of the Wild West. Decisions are frequently person-powered. Shots can come ringing out of nowhere, can ricochet, might be duds—anything is possible. What happens depends upon who shows up for the meeting—and part of what happens, and its predictability, depends upon whether those who show up have some understanding of the need for a truly evidence-based approach and if there is someone present who can help make that happen.

17. Product Decision-making Point #2: Physicians on the committee typically drive the decisions; however, if evidence-based practice is allowed to flourish, decision-making is likely to be based on the quality and usefulness of the evidence, decisions may be more predictable and objective, and decisions may be less person-powered and judgment-oriented.

18. Product Decision-making Point #3: Formulary decisions are usually comparative—at least in a broad sense. However, many groups utilize a class effect approach. This is irrespective of evidence-sophistication. We, however, believe that class effect may not be in the best interest of patients and can be particularly problematic when high quality science

with meaningful clinical outcomes becomes obscured or misappropriated because of this approach.

Now that we have given you greater insights into world of the customer and evidence, we want to help you better navigate this world.

COMMUNICATING WITH CUSTOMERS ABOUT MEDICAL EVIDENCE

Our objectives moving forward are to help you understand more about evidence issues important to customers, how to develop common ground over science and connect with customers over evidence. In this section, our discussion centers on these concepts—

1. Presentation of a step-wise approach for communicating about and connecting over evidence;

2. More on evidence quality issues;

3. Assessing customer approaches to evidence; and,

4. Practical guidance, advice, strategies, tips and efficiencies.

First, we will give you an overview of our prescription, if you will, for a roadmap for industry to best engage with customers over evidence, and then we will start filling in details.

A MAP OF THE 5 MILESTONES LEADING TO EFFECTIVE EVIDENCE COMMUNICATIONS WITH CUSTOMERS: RRAPP™

I. **Research ~ High Quality & Clinically Useful Evidence**
Conduct high-quality research on appropriate populations using good comparators and selecting useful endpoints that are meaningful to customers. Strive for solid research design and good execution, working to maximize good study performance outcomes and utilizing effective measurement methods.

II. **Report ~ Clarity & Transparency**
Provide transparent reporting that is meaningful to customers. Understand if there are any gaps between your research and its reporting and take steps to make needed information accessible.

III. **Appraise ~ Knowledge About The Evidence**
Apply critical appraisal skills to relevant research. This includes your own research and that of your competitors.

IV. **Prepare to Communicate About the Evidence ~ Know the Evidence Issues & Have Communication Aids**
Prepare for effective communications about evidence using all of the above. Be familiar with critically appraised information and typical issues

raised by customers. Have effective communication pieces, resources and options including education methods.

V. **Prepare to Connect Over the Evidence ~ Know the Customer to Interact with the Customer**
Apply skills for enhancing connecting over the evidence in your interactions with your specific customer in mind. This includes being able to assess your customer's climate for medical decision-making and their evidentiary knowledge and approach both organizationally and individually within the organization. This also includes being prepared to bridge gaps in evidentiary knowledge and skills. Have effective methods for addressing customers' questions.

RESEARCH ~ High Quality & Clinically Useful Evidence

Conduct high-quality research on appropriate populations using good comparators and selecting useful endpoints that are meaningful to customers. Strive for solid research design and good execution, working to maximize good study performance outcomes and utilizing effective measurement methods.

You may think your research is of the highest quality and it may be—we and others will be very happy about that. Unfortunately, much high quality research is obscured by lack of transparent reporting. But setting that aside for the moment, as we have pointed out, there is a large amount of research, published in even the best journals, that has sufficient study bias—such as lack of effective blinding—or risk of chance effects that the results cannot be relied upon. Also, there is a large amount of research that does not result in meaningful clinical benefit or is of uncertain benefit. Clinical usefulness is a combination of a clinically meaningful outcome—meaning an outcome that is truly of benefit to patients—and the size of the study results.

Consequently, we have put together a section in **Appendix B** to elaborate on some research design and performance elements that many times are overlooked by researchers and authors of papers or are problematic to customers in some way. We highly recommend that **all readers** of this book—even those who are experienced scientists—review the appendices as there is a lot of useful information to be gleaned that can be of use in reporting results and working with customers (plus there are some *fascinating* stories). And you do not want to miss out on our discussion of the increasingly popular "**real world data**" universe.

Topics we expound upon in **Appendix B** are these—

1. "Appropriate populations" and why customers might not (and might not "unfairly") be accepting of your population for study;

2. Comparators and typical customer misunderstandings and frustrations;

3. Important issues regarding endpoints—determining if endpoints are clinically significant, problems with composite endpoints and, lastly, endpoints and other considerations in oncology studies since these are so unique;

4. Maximizing good study performance outcomes (e.g., successful blinding is an example of a "study performance outcome")—we include some fascinating stories (and scandalous ones at that) about problems with blinding and concealing the assignment of subjects to their study groups (and if that just sounded dry, the stories are not!)—and why stopping clinical trials early for benefit is problematic;

5. Effective measurement methods—and the potential to lose customers' trust, including how customers might automatically reject your results due to problematic definitions of success or failure; and,

6. "Real world data" and CER (comparative effectiveness research)—customers are clamoring for CER, and you want to understand how comparative effectiveness studies could hurt your product.

REPORT ~ Clarity & Transparency

Provide transparent reporting that is meaningful to customers. Understand if there are any gaps between your research and its reporting and take steps to make needed information accessible.

Again, we are all rooting for good research. As we stated earlier, we and other groups with strong evidology skills have estimated that 10% or less of published medical evidence can actually be utilized due to the problems of unreliability, uncertainty of reliability and/or insufficient clinical utility. And we think that this low percentage is due in large part to uncertainty of reliability **because of lack of completeness and transparency in reporting**.

Having met many industry scientists and having worked closely with industry to fill in reporting gaps, we believe that there is frequently much excellence in industry studies. But reporting is highly problematic. In working with industry, it has become clear to us that one of the reasons for the reporting problem is that many authors of papers do not understand what it is that end-users need to see to evaluate studies. (In part, this is because authors tend to be unaware that end-users frequently *will* be evaluating their studies.)

When made aware that many users will be doing a critical appraisal of their studies and require more information, scientists have also told us that frequently editors call for them to cut methods and expand the discussion. And, in all likelihood, this comes about because editors of publications do not understand what it is that end-users need to see to evaluate studies. (And again, in part, this is because many editors tend to be unaware that end-users frequently *will* be evaluating studies—and this is frequently because editors, *too*, often lack critical appraisal skills and the awareness of the importance of critical appraisal.)

However, the good news is that often what we need to see in reporting can be expressed very succinctly, or additional information can be made available in an online appendix. If using an online source, however, be sure to make it very easy for the end user to find and access the information, including putting information in the publication as to where the information can be obtained.

Also, be aware that more sophisticated reviewers will not be content with being directed to information in the protocol without some kind of confirmation of what actually transpired. Studies have shown that oftentimes protocols are changed or not adhered to [Chan 08, Pildal 05]. Therefore, it is important to follow up with information that the protocol was not changed or to identify what was actually done in the study.

CONSORT, which stands for Consolidated Standards Of Reporting Trials, is a series of initiatives developed by various experts including scientists and journal editors in an attempt to improve reporting of clinical trials. Their main output has been the CONSORT Statement, which is a set of research reporting standards. Their website where you can find the Statement is http://www.consort-statement.org/.

We have taken the CONSORT document and annotated it to provide suggestions for what critical appraisers may be looking for in trial reporting. Because the CONSORT statement is primarily aimed at improving the quality of reporting of efficacy in superiority trials, extensions have been periodically issued, (e.g., regarding adverse events, non-inferiority and equivalence trials, pragmatic trials, etc.). Where we thought important, we have also included information from these extensions. **Our annotated version of the CONSORT Statement** is available at the **Reader Resource** web page, the URL for which is available at the end of part 1 of this book.

Our Reporting Ideals for Clinical Trials

In **Appendix C**, we present our general ideals in a framework of how we think of the stages of a clinical trial when we are assessing its validity. **Notice that we just said "our ideals."** Our ideals are in keeping with those of other evidence-savvy groups such as Cochrane, the CONSORT Group and others including evidence-sophisticated customers. **However, for clarity, because many customers are *not* familiar with these ideas, we take a shift in perspective in this section to say "we look for" instead of "customers look for..." to give you the most helpful information.**

You will want to pay close attention to these ideal reporting requirements for several reasons: 1) you want to know that your reporting is the best that it can be; 2) you want to know what many customers and other end-users of your publications and other information sources may be looking for; 3) you want to know what we train customers to look for when evaluating the quality of a study and its clinical usefulness; and, 4) your understanding of these ideals can give you an edge and flexibility in communications—both in planned structured pieces and in oral communications with customers.

Important: it is not our intent to list here everything that we consider in a critical appraisal, but rather to inform you of the kinds of information we and others may be interested in that helps us with our critical appraisal evaluations. We elaborate on **some** of these elements in **Appendix C,** and **Appendix F is our complete "SHORT CRITICAL APPRAISAL CHECKLIST—INTERVENTIONS FOR PREVENTION, SCREENING & THERAPY."** We have favored inclusion of items that are frequently omitted from publications or are worth discussing. However, an omission of an item from this list should not be taken to mean that we and other reviewers are not interested in information about that element.

And speaking of omissions, here is a reminder that when key information is omitted from a publication of a study, **that omission goes on our list of threats to validity because of our uncertainty about risk of bias.** This is a common approach utilized by many critical appraisers.

In **Appendix C**, we elaborate on ideal reporting recommendations for the following topics—

- Subject selection including **concise** ways to report how patients were allocated to their study groups and why this is critically important information;

- Study performance including advice on tagging outcomes in useful ways for appraisers, tips for presenting key information about blinding, why it is not wise to "test the success of blinding" and key information that should be reported for co-interventions to lessen the chance of your study being rejected;

- Data collection & loss of data—many customers will reject a study outright if attrition is high—factors which may reduce this possibility;

- Assessing the differences in outcomes in the study groups including transparency in detailing subject disposition (and why this can help your study if you have significant attrition), desirable population analysis methods and desirability in results reporting (how to make customers unhappy and how to make them happy and save them work);

- Non-inferiority and equivalence designs;

- Reporting of crossover trials;

- Protocol compliance;

- Diagnostic testing; and,

- Screening.

In short, it is important to report on anything that helps reviewers assess internal validity, clinical usefulness and external validity.

These are our tips for effective and transparent reporting—

1. Gain familiarity with reporting ideals (e.g., the suggestions listed here, Delfini Annotated Guide to CONSORT, our short critical appraisal checklist at **Appendix F**, The Cochrane Collaboration Handbook [Higgins 11], etc.);

2. Check studies against checklists for best critical appraisal practices and assume that your readers will include skilled critical appraisers;

3. Hone succinct descriptions for study design and for key elements in the 4 stages of a study (selection, performance, data collection/attrition and assessment);

4. Develop strategies for when editors get in the way of effective reporting (e.g., online appendices, communication pieces, dossiers, working with information partners such as ourselves or other vendors who can help you, etc.). It may

prove useful to have a conversation with an evidologist or someone else who is expert in critical appraisal before discussing your study with an editor.

5. Be aware that reporting gaps may have impact beyond customers that affect customer decisions (e.g., systematic reviews by Cochrane, ourselves and others who may be influential, write papers or otherwise work with customers and clinicians)—therefore, be sure to make information available and accessible to all; and,

6. Develop meaningful, comprehensive, clear and understandable communication pieces.

APPRAISE ~ Knowledge About The Evidence

Apply critical appraisal skills to relevant research. This includes your own research and that of your competitors.

Without A Working Knowledge of Critical Appraisal, Most Studies Look "Okay"

For industry staff who are involved in the conduct or the reporting of research or those communicating with customers and clinicians, we believe there are many benefits in possessing basic critical appraisal skills. Lack these skills and you lack crucially important information.

Can you or your company's "first-impression" staff have an effective science-based discussion with your most evidence-sophisticated customer?

- What would happen if the terms "concealment of allocation" or "intention-to-treat analysis" came up in a discussion with a customer?

- What would happen if asked about censoring rules?

- How could you and others respond if facing questions about sensitivity analyses for non-completers?

Do you or your company's staff communicating with customers understand the strengths and weaknesses of your studies and those of your competitors' through the lens of the customer—especially one that is evidence-savvy?

Can you or any of your staff answering customer questions diagnose the reviewer's level of evidence-sophistication and be supple enough to tailor communications accordingly?

- Can you or your company's staff tell when someone knows a term, but not the concept (e.g., concealment of allocation versus blinding, power, overlapping confidence intervals, etc.)? These concepts are not hard to understand, but they are frequently misunderstood.

- Can you or your company's staff tell when your individual contact in an otherwise evidence-savvy organization lacks such knowledge?

- How would you or your staff or company colleagues handle these situations?

As we stated before, we think it's very important for industry staff to understand the strengths and weaknesses of their own studies as well as those of competitor studies. For staff involved in communicating with customers—

1. Your company is in the science business. Therefore, we believe that it behooves you and your company to have at least a general understanding of what constitutes study quality and usefulness. What you know may end up being the decisive factor in your product getting a fair and balanced review and potentially helping patients—not understanding what constitutes quality science can harm both your business and patients.

2. Currently we see many missed opportunities for improved reporting and improved communications, and we see huge waste even beyond the dollar (e.g. use of human subjects and exposure to risk, human time and energy, opportunity-costs, etc.).

3. Understanding critical appraisal can create a common ground around science which can enhance internal communications within your company, can help with identification of communication approaches and guide both internal and external activities.

4. Understanding critical appraisal can help best maximize current and future opportunities.

Ideally, all industry staff involved in scientific design and reporting and in communications with customers have mastery of basic critical appraisal concepts with emphasis on bias and chance, a few key basic statistics and the general understanding of a few key analysis methods.

Another important point is that much evidence falls into a "grey zone" with potential for reasonable, opposing conclusions about use of that evidence. Often, this grey zone is a result of uncertainty. The more you know about critical appraisal, you may help elevate a study out of the grey zone and into an appreciation of its quality and clinical usefulness.

There are many resources available to you to help you delve deeper in understanding critical appraisal, including many resources **freely available** at our website at www.delfini.org and our recommendations for further reading, including our short book, **BASICS FOR EVALUATING MEDICAL RESEARCH STUDIES: A Simplified Approach**

A Few Critical Appraisal Essentials & Some *Crucially* Important Points

A brief critical appraisal primer, at a very high level, is provided as **Appendix A**. Here are a few basic points of great importance—

When it comes to medical science, as evidence-based medicine practitioners, we have **three essential questions**:

1. Is it true? = validity.

2. Is it useful? = clinical usefulness.

3. Is it usable? = accessible and understandable.

When it comes to clinical trials for interventions, study results are explained by bias, chance or cause and effect (truth). Therefore, "internal validity" (closeness to truth in the context of the study) is assessed by evaluating whether bias or chance are likely to have distorted study results.

Important Reminder: Bias tends to favor the intervention of interest that is being studied. We have already shared with you that bias has been documented to distort results up to a relative 50% or more for many individual biases. We will elaborate on this in greater detail in **Appendix F**, and there we will also elaborate on the evidence on the "uncertain risk of bias story" that we alluded to at the start of this book, providing greater detail about the Cochrane study.

Also, a reminder that clinical usefulness is a combination of the size of study results and the clinical meaningfulness of an outcome to a patient. The clinically meaningful outcomes are 1) morbidity; 2) mortality; 3) symptom relief; 4) physical, mental or emotional functioning; and, 5) health-related quality of life). Any other topic is an intermediate marker and requires a causal "proof of evidence" chain. How large an outcome must be to achieve meaningful clinical benefit is a judgment—different users will make different judgments, and often this is driven by context such as taking a population versus an individual patient's perspective.

"External validity" is closeness to truth outside of the study context in the "real world" circumstances of application of the intervention.

Know Your Studies; Know Your Competitors' Studies

Here is our key advice—

1. Ensure that you have some level of critical appraisal knowledge—the more, the better.

2. Know the strengths and limitations of your own and competitor studies. In other words, critically appraise these studies or have them critically appraised.

Having said that—

A Few Critical Appraisal Advisements

Be aware of several important things about critical appraisal—

1. Critical appraisal work is complex: there is no such thing as "perfection," and "exactitude" is not possible—although many people, wrongly, think that the application of medical science is more exacting than it really can be. There are good reasons why we frequently say "closeness to truth" as a definition for "internal validity."

3. The question framed by the reviewer will drive the review.

4. We cannot emphasize enough that the critical appraisal process is one of "discovery." Skills and insights vary greatly between critical appraisers, and much judgment is required. Critical appraisers with the same training may come to different conclusions—reasonably or due to variations in skills and understanding. Because **critical appraisal is inexact and a process of discovery**, not all potential issues may be identified in a review. This has very important implications for everyone in your organization who comes in contact with customers to discuss evidence.

5. Again, much research lands in a "grey-zone" with potential for reasonable, opposing conclusions.

6. There are frequently exceptions to critical appraisal "norms" because of contextual issues in trials. Be aware that many times the most correct answer to any generic critical appraisal question is, "It depends..." For example, larger rates of loss of data or subjects may be accepted by some customers if the attrition is judged to not disrupt the balance (similar prognostic factors) in the study groups.

A reminder that our short critical appraisal checklist is included as **Appendix F**.

PREPARE TO COMMUNICATE ABOUT EVIDENCE ~ Know the Evidence Issues & Have Communication Aids

Prepare for effective communications about evidence using all of the above. Be familiar with critically appraised information and typical issues raised by customers. Have effective communication pieces, resources and options including education methods.

Preparing for effective communications about evidence entails familiarity with relevant research, anticipation of issues that a customer might raise or need addressed in some way and the development of ways to address those issues.

Here is our key advice—

1. Be familiar with the critical appraisal findings of your studies and those of your competitors.

2. Be familiar with any reporting gaps in your research and identify ways to address those gaps.

3. Use this information to create effective communication pieces and resources.

4. Prepare strategies to deal with errors, misconceptions and thinking that is off-the-mark. Prepare methods for just-in-time education, if needed, both on specific studies and about critical appraisal in general. Sometimes a little education can go a long way toward product approval or keeping a product covered.

We recommend creating a well-documented critical appraisal report in two ways— one which can be shared with a customer and a second that includes "advisories" or educational commentaries for your company staff. This report can be structured to list the critical appraisal item, critical appraisal findings and, for internal staff, other information to help them plan their communications with individual customers. Below is an example to show you how this might look for a single critical appraisal item—study size.

Critical Appraisal Example with Industry Advisements—

Critical Appraisal Area of Consideration: Selection Bias

Number of Study Participants

- Critical Appraisal Findings: 1199 randomized patients = large study size

---

Comments for Internal Industry Staff

- Large population for study is a good study factor.

Key Points About Study Size

1. Small studies are those with a study sample of 100 or less.
2. Small studies are more prone to chance effects and lack generalizability.
3. Our study would be considered large, which is a strength.

Key Points About Customers

1. Some customers are confused about power and may look at the power calculation and believe that "power was not reached" if fewer patients completed the study than estimated for the power calculation. These customers should be advised that the purpose of a power calculation is to guestimate the number of patients that need to be enrolled in a study. The answer as to whether a study was sufficiently powered lies in the results. Power means that a sufficient number of patients were studied to find a statistically significant outcome, if one exists.

2. In our study, statistically significant outcomes occurred—therefore, these outcomes were sufficiently powered.

To give you a closer look at how this report can be prepared, an example of a critical appraisal of a real study with evidence advisements that we have prepared is available at the online **Reader Resource** web page.

Anticipate questions and have answers ready up-front to proactively address gaps in the reporting of your research and any areas in your research that could be considered to be in the "grey zone." Having a working understanding of your research and of your competitors' studies will help you anticipate customer questions. Here's a sample list of the kinds of questions that we have heard customers ask.

Sample Issues Customers May Raise (whether they are legitimate concerns or correct in their understanding or not)

The population—

1. The studied population is not like ours. Please explain.

2. There are no details about generation of the randomization sequence or concealment of allocation to study groups—what did you do?

3. The population studied is very heterogeneous. Did you analyze pre-specified subgroups, and what were the outcomes?

The primary outcome measure—

4. Is a surrogate measure. You will need to make the case for the clinical relevance of outcome X.

5. Is a composite measure. Justify your choices.

Performance issues—

6. We need details of blinding; how was blinding accomplished? What is the likelihood of successful blinding?

7. How did you blind subjects and cross-over points?

8. You provided insufficient information about co-interventions. How do the groups compare?

Attrition—

9. In many studies we are not provided complete information on how many people were lost to follow-up, and we want to know how many, when and why.

10. How do you explain the greater (withdrawals/ protocol violations / losses to follow-up / fill-in-the-blank) between the studied groups?

Analysis—

11. We need more detailed information about your Kaplan-Meier analyses—who was censored, why were they censored, when, how do they compare to others?

12. Were the baseline characteristics of the completers similar in both groups and to the originally randomized group?

13. What were your imputation methods for missing data? Is there a sensitivity analysis?

14. LOCF is prone to bias; did you do confirmatory analyses?

15. How did you avoid double-counting in your composite endpoint?

16. What is driving the composite? We want to see reporting of individual outcome components.

17. How do you justify stopping early for efficacy?

18. Your primary outcome did not reach significance—why should we accept the secondary outcomes?

19. You are claiming superiority, but this was a non-inferiority design. Explain.

20. Defend the appropriateness of your delta in non-inferiority and equivalence trials.

Important: Again, if you note that key information is not available in the publication, find a way to make that information available and make it easily accessible to any end-user—not just customers. Customers may rely upon a critical appraisal or other information prepared by people like us—and if we can't easily find and access your information, you may miss an important opportunity that might otherwise give your product a fair and balanced review and help patients.

To help you prepare for just-in-time education about critical appraisal, in the **appendices** we provide you with details of key areas of frequent misunderstanding by customers which you can use to help create general educational moments. A wealth of freely available information can help you with this step at www.delfini.org and at the **Reader Resource** web page.

Sample Ways to Convey Evidence-based Information

The critical appraisal example at the **Reader Resource** web page can give you access to a wealth of ideas including the format we use when we do these reviews and how we report on key critical appraisal elements. You can study the customer advisements in this case example, and you will see our approach to providing a strong rationale and making the case for study reliability and usefulness of study results.

As evidence-based clinical improvement experts, our interest is ultimately in medical decision-making and, therefore, we have a strong interest in decision-support including decision aids, information aids and action aids. This topic is beyond the scope of this book; however, we have included a couple of URLs below to some decision-support examples available on our website which are accessible from the **Reader Resource** web page as are most of the other URLs listed in this book:

www.delfini.org/page_SamePage_RxMessagingScripts.htm; and,

www.delfini.org/Delfini_Semaphore_Tool_HYPOTHETICAL.pdf

PREPARE TO CONNECT OVER THE EVIDENCE ~ Know the Customer to Interact with the Customer

Apply skills for enhancing connecting over the evidence in your interactions with your specific customer in mind. This includes being able to assess your customer's climate for medical decision-making and evidentiary knowledge and approach both organizationally and individually within the organization. This also includes being prepared to bridge gaps in evidentiary knowledge and skills. Have effective methods for addressing customers' questions.

Here is our advice—

1. You want to understand the customer's business model, company and customer leadership perspectives, company priorities for triangulation issues, staff orientation and recommendations, and decision-making committee operation and dynamics. And you want to understand their approach to the evidence. This combination may help you understand if and how the evidence will be used, along with other factors likely to affect decisions.

2. Know how to judge evidence-sophistication of customers and your colleagues who may interact with them.

3. Know effective ways to answer customers' evidence questions.

A key point about connecting with your customers—and now more than ever before—is that you might get only one chance to connect with them. Again, this is a very strong reason for ensuring at least basic critical appraisal skills for you and all of your company's staff who communicate with customers.

Where the evidence is sound, evidence tends to be a neutralizing force if you can create engagement over the evidence by awareness, information, logic, clarity and transparency. That is because evidence is more objective than opinion, and solid evidence coming from high quality studies where there is meaningful clinical benefit may speak for itself. We have seen this over and over again in committee and project team processes where attention to the evidence in a clear fashion has unified people when they are focused on patients. And focusing on solid and clinically meaningful evidence can build trust.

In addition to what we have already covered above, here are some more tips—

1. Be mindful that you may get only one or a limited number of opportunities to communicate about your science.

2. Try and think with the lens of the customer. What are their obligations, needs and requirements, etc.? What are their driving forces, and what are their restraining forces? When it comes to the evidence, how can you make their review easier for them?

3. When it comes to approaches to evidence, what are you dealing with organizationally and who are you dealing with individually? Differentiate between what the organizational reputation is with respect to an evidence-based approach and who is actually working on a review of your product. Usually, that person will end up being the key communicator of the evidence to others. Where is he or she on the evidence-based awareness and knowledge continuum? If in a meeting, who is the Alpha communicator in the room? Is someone else present whom you really have to address? Where are the key people you are talking to on the evidence-sophistication spectrum?

Impressionistically, here is what we see on a rough scale of 1 to 10 in terms of understanding critical appraisal principles and their application:

1—2: I trust the FDA. I know I need randomized controlled trials (RCTs) for supporting claims of efficacy, but that's all I really know (and some customers don't even know that). Given this, I pretty much accept all evidence.

3—4: I suspect that I need to engage with evidence differently. But I don't know what I don't know. I have uncertainty, discomfort and suspicions. But because I don't know enough, I live with discomfort and feel stuck in the *status quo*. It makes me edgy and mistrustful.

5—8: I have modest to fair to strong critical appraisal skills. I may have some misunderstandings. I may misapply some of the principles. I may rely more on the concepts than on the context of the study. (Note that with some people in this group, there is a risk of misunderstanding or misapplication of the concepts or there may be a lack of critical thinking being applied.)

9—10: I have strong skills in critical appraisal. I critically think through context. My focus is on **the likely impact** of bias and chance on study results. (Note that this latter approach frequently takes a lot of time.)

There are several things that have impact on where a person or an organization may be on this scale. Drivers toward number 10 start with awareness. This cannot be overstated in a world where so many professionals who are engaged in health care decision-making have zero to little understanding of the issues with medical science and what constitutes valid science. When you have individuals and organizations that have this awareness, then the next key driver on the continuum is whether they have a commitment to an effective evidence-based approach.

And then, as is true about so much in our universe, the buck stops there. Literally. You can have very knowledgeable individuals with a strong commitment to evidence-based practice, but without an investment in such an approach, critical assessment of the evidence falls to the wayside. And the investment is usually fairly steep. Performing critical appraisal effectively is labor-intensive. However, if it is not done at all or if it is done fairly poorly, we all lose.

So to recomb this slightly differently, drivers toward evidence-based practice are awareness, commitment and investment. Barriers against evidence-based practice are lack of awareness, lack of skills, dollars and time (the latter two of which are sometimes, but not always, related).

Keep in mind that even the evidence-savvy may have evidentiary misunderstandings—we all do. Also keep in mind that even those who are evidence-savvy may have major time issues which may get in their way of doing a more comprehensive review.

4. As teachers, we get some crazy questions (and we mean this with no disrespect; what we mean by this is that crossed wires, misunderstandings and confusions can sometimes make it really hard to figure out if a question even makes sense or where someone is on Planet Evidence—so more than anything, this is an awareness-raising comment that this is likely to happen to you too). Be prepared to do a little critical appraisal education, if you can. When we get a question that seems very off or hard to detangle, we try to get the questioner to step away from the question and say, "Let's review the basics." That often helps to get everyone on track.

5. Where are they on the evidence-acceptance spectrum for your research? Where are they with a decision for your product? What are their barriers, doubts and questions? You want to discover their story, and you want to diagnose and discover the key contextual elements of that story. To do this, you want to do a lot of listening with little interrupting and gather information as you go. Are they too "shy" or uncomfortable to admit it's really all about cost? Be encouraging that they cleanly address issues about the evidence first—this is most fair and the right thing for patient care.

If your evidence is sufficient and benefits outweigh harms, it is highly likely that your therapy will be considered in the context of other "non-evidentary" factors such as currently available options or cost.

If your evidence is insufficient or borderline, and benefits outweigh harms, it is still possible that your therapy will be considered against other factors *unless* alternatives are looked at more favorably because of their evidence or because of a decision to accept standards or generics without further evidence review.

6. A decision point of "uncertainty" may give you an opportunity for further discussion as might a decision point of "no." Again, there are many reasons that go into a coverage decision as we described earlier in **A Framework for Medical Coverage Decision-Making: A Sampling of Decision Consideration.**

Prepare to Assess an Organization's Approach to Understanding and Utilizing Evidence: Tips

The starting point for understanding your contact's placement on the evidence-based knowledge continuum is to first gain clarity about what is really going on in his or her organization with respect to evidence-based practice. For a long time now, EBM has been a popular buzzword. Everybody wants to say that they're taking an evidence-based approach, but in fact many do not know what that really means. A lot of people mistake selecting supporting references for evidence-based practice, but that is what EBM leader, Dr. David Eddy, refers to as "evidence sprinkling." Many monographs and study reviews do not reflect true evidence evaluation at all, but can be likened more to book reports.

Here are what we consider to be **the hallmarks of evidence-based medicine**:

1. When seeking information on a topic, a systematic search is conducted for science and science-based information using evidence-based searching and filtering techniques. "Applying a systematic search" means a search that includes utilization of the National Library of Medicine, which is accessed through the online PubMed database. "Systematic search" also means that all relevant and potentially useful studies are accessed, rather than studies being "cherry-picked." Focusing solely on interventional research, it is an industry standard that evidence-based searching and filtering techniques allow for limiting studies accessed to randomized controlled trials (RCTs). However, additional searches may be undertaken for observational studies and other information about safety.

2. All sources of information to guide medical decision-making are critically appraised, using science-based principles, for validity and usefulness. Again, staff skills and allotted time make or break how effectively this is done.

3. Methods used and reporting are transparent so that the work can be evaluated for quality and can be replicated and updated.

4. Wording of any conclusions drawn from the science is carefully crafted to be as valid as possible.

5. Clinical information sources are updated when significant new information becomes available, and such information is periodically sought.

As part of your research into the organization's evidence commitment, sophistication and approach, important questions to get answered include whether or not the organization has a formal method for evaluating interventions. If yes, you will want to gain an understanding of the **specifics of their processes.**

1. Do they take a class effect approach?

2. How do they determine which studies will be evaluated?

3. How do they prioritize their reviews or decide which class of drugs to review and how often to review them? Is their decision based on safety, cost, clinical importance or efficacy and is one weighted heavier than others? Or is it based on cost solely or just provider requests, etc.

4. How do they conduct critical appraisals? Do they have criteria? What are those criteria? Do they utilize a documented, standard approach such as using a form or a checklist or some template? What are the items on that document? Do they apply standards to rank threats to validity, or is their review contextually based and dependent upon the unique aspects of the studies? Some standards may be reasonable, but staff who have strong critical appraisal skills and base their reviews on contextual considerations of studies are likely to do a better and more fair job of critical appraisal. How many people are involved in a review? An appraisal that does not include multiple appraisers or some kind of peer review process is likely to be weaker. Are they willing to share their reviews with you?

5. How does the organization ensure that staff have adequate critical appraisal skills? Because so few health care professionals involved in medical decision-making have received training in critical appraisal or possess these skills, an organization that does not address this in some way is likely to have staff involved in reviews who are not truly doing critical appraisal or who are doing it poorly.

6. Another important factor to understand is the culture for clinical decision-making and whether the staffers truly do or do not affect formulary decisions. So a worthwhile question to ask is, "What percentage of the time are recommendations of staffers accepted?" Other ways to ask about this and gain additional information is to inquire about what happens in committee meetings when clinicians disagree or ignore the evidence-based assessments of staffers or whether staffers feel comfortable communicating about their reviews during the discussions?

The goal of these inquiries is to determine whether there is trust and acceptance of staffers' reviews or whether there is a chasm between staffer presentations and documents and decision-maker deliberations and decision-making. This is not to say that staffers' recommendations should always be accepted. There are many reasons that go into accepting an intervention for coverage. The key here is how likely is it that a staffer's evidence-based review will be accepted—or is the likely reality that any evidence review work is going to be disregarded as if it had never been done?

Keep in mind that gaining clarity about whether or not an organization is actually performing in an evidence-based fashion may frequently be challenging because of the use of buzzwords and because of the frequent problem of people not knowing what they don't know in this area. Therefore, the more details you can gain access to, the greater your insights are likely to be, provided that you have a reasonable understanding of what constitutes an evidence-based approach and at least a basic familiarity with critical appraisal concepts.

Prepare to Assess an Individual's Approach to Understanding and Utilizing Evidence: Tips

In addition to understanding an organization's approach to the evidence, you will also want to understand the approach and the skill level of the individuals engaged in the evidence-based work. Even if an organization lacks a commitment to an EBM approach, it may be the case that a staff person involved in interventional reviews does, in fact, possess critical appraisal skills. Possessing those skills, however, is not the same as applying them. Even if the staff person does have such skills, if the organization is not providing support (e.g., time), it is unlikely that the individual would be able to conduct a very thorough evidence-based review.

Conversely, just because an organization expresses commitment to an EBM approach and even can tell you how they ensure that staff are skilled in critical appraisal, a review of your intervention may still be in the hands of someone who is not very skilled at all.

The best way to understand an individual's approach to utilizing evidence is to be familiar with critical appraisal concepts and then engage him or her in a conversation, discussing concepts in general or the specifics of his or her review of the studies of your intervention of interest. Keep in mind, however, that because there are no standards in education or testing for critical appraisal, a person may have very sophisticated knowledge of some of the concepts and have incomplete or incorrect knowledge of others. In this latter case, it is possible that only by working with such an individual over time that you will be able to gauge the extent of his or her general knowledge.

The potential for how bias might impact study results is usually very logical. Therefore, people who truly understand bias in clinical trials should generally be able to explain the import of various biases in jargon-free ways that you can understand. If they do a good job of this, then they probably have good critical appraisal skills, at least in those areas they can simply and clearly explain.

Prepare to Assess an Organization's and/or an Individual's Evidence-sophistication: Sample Questions

Here are some sample questions, the answers to which can be useful to you in several ways—not only in understanding evidence-sophistication, but also including understanding reporting requirements of individual customers and their critical appraisal staff. As we've explained, one of the great frustrations expressed by many customers who work closely with evidence is that often reporting of study methods and execution is lacking in the publication. By better understanding reviewer requirements, you can help improve reporting directly, if that is your role, or indirectly by conveying this information to the appropriate people in your company, and you can be more proactive in finding answers when information is otherwise missing in the publication.

We will discuss typical missed reporting requirements and needs in greater detail in **Appendix B**, but here are some questions that potentially can give you a little biopsy of the approach of the individual or the organization. **This list is not a complete list of key critical appraisal considerations**. For that information, see **Appendix F** for our short critical appraisal checklist. **We have selected the following questions for this section because they are answerable in general ways, are meaningful and/or represent areas of frequent misunderstanding or ignorance.**

In **Appendix D**, we will discuss the rationale for including each question along with some descriptive information and considerations. For instances in which there are frequent misunderstandings, this information may help you provide additional education on specific areas affecting a review of your science. We have seen important decisions change when such important information regarding the validity of a study is brought to light.

1. How do they identify studies for review? (And how their selection of studies could be detrimental to a favorable product.)

2. How do they conduct a review?

3. What weight do they put on blinding? (And why they should put a lot of weight on blinding.)

4. How do they evaluate the use of co-interventions?

5. How do they evaluate placebo effect?

6. How do they evaluate power? (And do they really know what this means? Frequently not...)

7. How do they approach attrition? (Why their approach could be wrongly hurtful to your product.)

8. How do they evaluate intention–to–treat analyses? (And are you reporting on these correctly or incorrectly—roughly half of investigators fall into the latter group.)

9. How do they evaluate time-to-event analyses?

10. What is their process for evaluating clinical significance?

11. How do they utilize confidence intervals? (And how a common misconception can result in a mistaken interpretation of your product's results when compared to a competitor's.)

12. Do they have special considerations for handling secondary outcomes? (Potential for HUGE problems for you if you have statistically significant secondary outcomes, but your primary outcomes are non-significant. Many customers will reject your study outright. Is this fair? And can this be overcome?)

13. What is their approach to all-or-none results? (And what are all-or-none results?)

14. What are their considerations for evaluating non-inferiority and equivalence?

15. Do they accept claims of superiority in a non-inferiority or equivalence design? (Potential for HUGE problems for you if you have statistically significant outcomes using one of these types of comparative designs—but the customer may not accept this outcome. Is this fair? And can this be overcome? The answer is a solid, "yes.")

16. What is their approach to secondary studies or sources such as systematic reviews, clinical guidelines, compendia, comparative effectiveness research and health care economic studies?

17. What is their knowledge of the clinical disease state targeted by your product? This is important both from an organizational standpoint and with respect to the individuals reviewing your product. Do they understand special aspects of the disease that are important in treatment decisions? (Make no assumptions—you can really get hurt on this one—and patients may lose out on effective solutions due to misunderstandings.)

18. How do they evaluate safety?

19. How do they conduct reviews of studies of diagnostic tests and screening?

For elaborations on these questions and details, see **Appendix D.**

Preparing Answers to Customers' Questions

We have both worked with customers to evaluate industry responses to their questions, and we have worked with industry to help respond to customer requests. In general, we have observed that industry staff often miss the point of the question, get overly elaborate with minutiae that only tends to confuse things and miss opportunities when customer questions have missed the mark. When responding to requests, our general advice is—

1. Questions will frequently be about studies considered by appraisers to be in the "grey or borderline" area for validity. More than one answer may be correct. Therefore, maximize your opportunity to address concerns by being aware of this so that you don't go down just one path if another should have been taken.

2. If you can, try to get clarity about what is really being asked. For example, a customer who is asking for elaborations on attrition details is possibly focused on the effect of attrition on reported results. Or they may be concerned about a change in the studied population that may affect generalizability to their population. What are they really trying to understand? It is a fairly safe bet that evidence-savvy customers will ask questions that fall into one or more of the following areas: study design, selection bias, performance bias, data collection/attrition bias, assessment bias, chance and clinical usefulness. Optimal preparation to address questions requires knowledge of what the above issues are generally all about, their potential impacts on reliability and relevance and how they are assessed—including how they are sometimes assessed incorrectly by customers and being prepared to educate on what is actually correct.

3. If you cannot get further clarity about what they are asking directly, what do you think are the possible issues? If you are working with evidence-savvy groups (or physicians, whether evidence-savvy or not), it is not likely that they are concerned with pharmacology issues, so don't overwhelm them with a lot of unnecessary detail and take up precious time with that kind of information. The occasional pharmacist may become enrapt with a "beautiful molecule," but doctors do not and are the chief decision-makers of customer committees—and evidence-savvy pharmacists know that is not what they really should be focusing on. Companies spend way too much time in this arena, and generally it is just not helpful.

Our advice is to look to critical appraisal issues, searching for threats to validity due to bias and chance, and also focus on potential concerns about clinical usefulness. This approach can be of benefit even with customers who understand little about critical appraisal if your studies are done well and your results are good.

Also, when looking at clinical usefulness, pay close attention to the evidence on burden of illness. We are not talking about "disease-mongering." We have seen instances where companies have not done sufficient work to show valid and meaningful evidence on impact to patients, and we've been able to help by building an evidence-based chain of proof to help payers and health systems better understand their *own* customer base ("the patient") and his or her needs. We have already advised you that an important question to get answered of your customer contact is, "What is their knowledge of the clinical disease state targeted by your product?" Again, this is important both from an organizational standpoint and with respect to the individuals reviewing your product. Sometimes there will be a big gap. Also, because of concerns about disease-mongering practices and marketing practices in general, suspicions in this area run high. So when burdens to patients are truly missed, a transparent and well-done evidence-based approach is very important for patient care.

Lastly, consider issues of external validity. Be aware that this area is judgment laden and harder to address. If the available evidence pertains to a population quite different from your customer's population, judgement will be needed to project outcomes for the customer's population.

4. Answer the question directly AND address what you believe to be the actual issue or issues.

5. Be knowledgeable about the study protocol and whether any changes have taken place. If so, why were the changes made? What was actually done?

6. Succinct may be sufficient. Again, we see much unnecessary and frequently distracting information which bogs the reviewer down and sometimes leads to further confusion—especially when the information doesn't relate to what is being asked. Further confusion may lead to a door being slammed shut—or it may lead to other questions that just create greater complications and more noise and less clarity.

We advise seeking being "complete enough." In saying this we are not advocating lack of transparency. We are advocating thoughtful disclosure of that which is meaningful and useful for evaluating internal validty, clinical usefulness, external validity and the disclosure of any other meaningful information that can be helpful to a customer for medical decision-making such as pertinent information helping to evaluate any triangulation issues.

7. If a question reveals a misunderstood area, use that as an opportunity to nicely educate on an evidence-based principle. Some frequent misunderstandings on the part of customers include—

- Use of observational studies;

- Power;

- Concealment of allocation (versus blinding);

- Attrition (not necessarily understanding the real issues);

- Lack of understanding of issues in subgroup analyses (e.g., concluding no benefit in a subpopulation when the study is not powered to do so—meaning an insufficient number of people to show a difference between groups when one, in fact, exists and would be discoverable with more people);

- Overlapping confidence intervals; and,

- Determining superiority from non-inferiority or equivalence trials (yes, it is okay to do this—though many customers mistakenly think it is not).

We are now ready to take you on a more detailed dive into selected parts and pieces. But first, we want to give you a quick summation of where we have been and where we are going.

SUMMARY OF PART 1

Again, we have organized this book in **two parts** which are equally important. The first part of this book—which you have just completed—is meant to provide you with general information. Many more elaborations, details examples and stories are available to you in the **Appendices** immediately following **About the Authors** which we encourage you to read whether you possess strong scientific skills or not. For example, we elaborate on the questions that we have shared with you for assessing an organization and an individual's evidence sophistication. We also include an example of what a critical appraisal looks like and much more.

Overall, our suggestions to you are detailed in our RRAPP™ prescription for you of the map of the 5 milestones leading to effective evidence communication with customer. In brief—

1. Understand how customers may view and use evidence.

2. Fit research design to the needs of customers, clinicians and other medical decision-makers and ensure reporting to enable critical appraisal.

3. Understand critical appraisal—the basics at a minimum, but preferably in depth.

4. Understand applicable strengths and limitations of the research for your products and those of your competitors.

5. Understand how to use the evidence to support decisions and to inform communications with customers, maximizing the value of your contact time.

6. Understand how to connect with customers over evidence.

We hope that the information provided in this book will improve understanding of the important link between quality of medical evidence and reliability of reported study results—and how customers, health care providers and other medical decision-makers are increasingly aware of this. Much evidence is not reliable or is of uncertain reliability and clinical usefulness—and frequently this is due to lack of sufficient reporting of important study reliability elements. **This makes it impossible to accurately anticipate what benefits and harms patients are likely to experience with interventions**—and decision-makers are, at best, reluctant to support the use of interventions that have not demonstrated their value.

To determine reliability and clinical usefulness, knowledge of the important concepts and methods of critical appraisal are required along with clinical knowledge. Those who understand these concepts and their potential use in practice on the customer/provider side will possess enhanced understanding of reliability and usefulness and will be in a much stronger position to foster meaningful conversations about clinical trials and other medical evidence or to help ensure that they happen.

Although some physicians, pharmacists, nurses, epidemiologists and others do possess some critical appraisal skills, in many cases, skills are rudimentary or even less than that. In fact, our experience is that the majority of professional medical decision-makers are not well-equipped to critically appraise medical evidence. This means that many therapeutic decisions are made without knowledge of the quality of the evidence. Your understanding the concepts discussed here can potentially help to elevate their understanding, thereby helping to mitigate decisions made on unreliable information or on information that is not likely to be clinically useful.

Industry professionals involved in research and reporting must use critical appraisal knowledge to ensure adequate study design, conduct, reporting and communications about the evidence for a product to best help medical decision-makers. Transparency will become increasingly important as more health care professionals discover the importance of an evidence-based approach.

For those involved in communicating with customers, clinicians and other medical decision-makers, basic competency in understanding critical appraisal concepts is a foundational element in discerning where various customers are on the evidence-sophistication spectrum. Their position on this spectrum will affect customers' thinking and coverage decisions. With knowledge of what constitutes reliable and clinically useful science and how to conduct critical appraisals comes the ability to effectively converse about a myriad of important issues with customers who vary greatly in their own ability to evaluate medical science.

Ultimately, the patient is the one for whom value is the primary question. Understanding key critical appraisal concepts and their import by everyone involved in health care decision-making—from physicians to sales representatives, from scientists to customers—is doing right by patients—and which ultimately includes you, the reader, and your loved ones and friends. Ultimately, we are all patients, so ultimately we are all in this together.

For more details, see the **Reader Resource** web page and the **Appendices** which can be found *after* **About the Authors**.

READER RESOURCE WEB PAGE

For tools and online resources:
www.delfinigrouppublishing.com/ResourcesEBMIndustryGuide.htm

ABOUT THE AUTHORS

Delfini Group is a public service entrepreneurship founded to advance applied evidence- and value-based clinical quality improvements and methods through practice, training and facilitation. Much of Delfini's work is dedicated to help solve the little known societal problem of medical misinformation. Delfini has contributed to text books, advised government entities, worked with health care systems, customers and manufacturers and has trained thousands of health care professionals in evidence-based quality improvement.

Michael E. Stuart MD & Sheri Ann Strite are medical information scientists, medical evidologists and evidence-based clinical improvement experts. Mike and Sheri combine academic and practical experience to—

- Train people in how to evaluate medical research studies.
- Perform evidence reviews and systematic reviews.
- Help health care systems and others apply evidence- and value-based clinical quality improvement methods including special help for work groups such as clinical guideline development teams, pharmacy & therapeutics and medical technology assessment committees, clinical quality improvement teams, journal clubs and more.
- Train physicians and others in communicating with patients.

In addition, industry-centered experience includes—

1. Advising on study design.
2. Assisting with sensitivity analyses.
3. Analyzing research and providing advice for reporting, decision-aids and communications with customers.
4. Assisting in responding to customer queries about research and clinical issues such as case-building for burden of illness.
5. Content development including developing clinical recommendations, practice guidelines and pathways.
6. Developing performance measures.
7. Assisting with appropriate application of real world data and comparative effectiveness research (CER).
8. Economic modeling advisements.
9. Evidence-based medicine communications training.
10. Conducting programs for customers.
11. Facilitating clinical quality improvement projects.

Sheri Ann Strite, Co-founder, Principal & Managing Partner, initiated many Delfini health care improvement strategies, tools and training programs including the popular Delfini critical appraisal training program. Formerly she was Associate Director, Program Development, University of California, San Diego (UCSD) Family & Preventive Medicine, School of Medicine, where she taught faculty, physicians, residents, medical and pharmacy students and medical librarians. She was also a member of the UCSD Family Medicine Research Leaders and faculty for their Research Fellowship in the Department of Family & Preventive Medicine. Prior to UCSD, Ms. Strite worked in clinical improvement, education and research at Group Health Cooperative in Seattle, Washington, where she held various positions including leadership, research management and administration.

Michael E. Stuart MD, Co-founder, President & Medical Director, is a family physician and was appointed a clinical faculty position at the University of Washington in 1975. He is the former Director of the Department of Clinical Improvement and Education at Group Health Cooperative in Seattle, Washington, where he led development of more than 35 evidence-based clinical guidelines and other clinical improvements, chaired the Pharmacy & Therapeutics and Medical Technology Assessment Committees. His work has received praise from prominent health care leaders such as David Eddy MD, Don Berwick MD, Health Ministry of New Zealand and the US Navy Bureau of Medicine.

Topics upon which Delfini has written and taught include critical appraisal of medical literature, evidence-based committee processes, health care content development, technology assessment, population-based care, projecting economic and health outcomes, performance measurement, patient decision-making, facilitating provider behavior change, physician/patient communications, developing and implementing clinical guidelines, and creating information, decision and action aids for clinical care.

Strite and Stuart are authors of—

BASICS FOR EVALUATING MEDICAL RESEARCH STUDIES:
A Simplified Approach—And Why Your Patients Need You To Know This

Delfini Group Evidence-based Practice Series
Short How-to Guide Book

Available at—
http://www.delfinigrouppublishing.com/

Editorial Reviews for *Basics for Evaluating Medical Research Studies*:

"Highly recommended! Sheri and Mike have distilled their many years of hands-on experience evaluating medical research and teaching others to do so into a succinct, practical and easy-to-understand handbook that clearly and simply explains to readers how to assess the quality and usefulness of clinical trials and other medical articles. Key statistical concepts are presented clearly and explained in a math-free way that is not intimidating. They also equip readers with a wealth of practical tools that have been refined over time into 1-page guides and checklists which are used by many around the world." **John C. Pezzullo, PhD, Biostatistician and Author of *Biostatistics for Dummies***

"I am full of admiration for this terrific little book on evaluating medical research studies which is written clearly, simply and appropriately for a starter audience. Those with more experience often need reminding of the basics and can benefit from it too. I know of no other book that has succeeded so well in getting everything important covered so succinctly, which the authors have done brilliantly well." **Richard Lehman, MA, BM, BCh, MRCGP, Senior Research Fellow, Oxford, and Blogger, *BMJ Journal Watch***

"This book provides a great introduction and guide for anyone who wants to understand how to interpret clinical research but feels intimidated by science or statistics. Sheri and Mike transform their experience of teaching these concepts to thousands of people into a format like they are speaking to you directly. For the evidologist there is a nice compilation of the evidence for critical appraisal components."
Brian S. Alper, MD, MSPH, FAAFP, Editor-in-Chief, DynaMed (dynamed.ebscohost.com)

"This noteworthy book educates on many issues we address daily at **HealthNewsReview**.org. Written for physicians and other healthcare professionals, the authors write in terms the public can understand. Journalists who feed off a steady of diet of journal articles should read it along with the collection of tools at delfini.org. The book is only 112 pages. It won't overwhelm you, but will educate you on many of the themes we touch on so often as we analyze media messages about medical research studies. Strite and Stuart also provide examples to help educate." **Gary Schwitzer, Publisher, www.HealthNewsReview.org**

Available at—
http://www.delfinigrouppublishing.com/

PART 2: APPENDICES—MORE PRACTICAL HELP, ADVICE & TIPS
Elaborations, Details, More Stories from the Trenches and A Few
Technical Items

A descriptive list of the appendices follows to give you a flavor of what you will find in this second part of the book. However, even if you think you know a topic, **we encourage all readers to at least skim each of these sections.** You might think you know a topic represented well, but you might find a new way to teach or communicate something, gain a clarification, experience a surprise, run across an interesting story or example or find some other useful nugget of information.

Because some of these sections are elaborations on what we've just covered, **we may repeat some information from Part 1 in places for readability.**

DESCRIPTION OF THE APPENDICES

APPENDIX A: EBM TERMS FOR *EVERYONE*—A BRIEF ORIENTATION TO CRITICAL APPRAISAL

Even if you are well versed in critical appraisal, you might find this section helpful to establish common ground with customers—even Mars and Venus need a common language to communicate. This appendix provides a few more details about critical appraisal including some examples. However, this appendix only provides a satellite view and does not provide instruction about doing the actual work of critical appraisal.

APPENDICES FOR OUR PRESCRIPTION: A MAP OF THE 5 MILESTONES LEADING TO EFFECTIVE EVIDENCE COMMUNICATIONS WITH CUSTOMERS—RRAPP™

This appendix provides elaborations and details for 3 of the 5 milestones on the journey to effective EBM communications.

APPENDIX B: RESEARCH ~ High Quality & Clinically Useful Evidence—DETAILS

Here we elaborate upon **selected** study design and performance elements, some of which are of special concern to customers and one of which is subject to frequent misunderstanding—and that is the very unique world of "real world data."

APPENDIX C: REPORT ~ Clarity & Transparency—DETAILS

In this appendix, we elaborate upon selected ideals for study reporting.

APPENDIX D: PREPARE TO CONNECT OVER THE EVIDENCE ~ Know the Customer to Interact with the Customer—DETAILS

In this section, we flesh out questions for assessing the evidence sophistication of organizations and individuals.

APPENDIX E: RISK OF BIAS DETAILS

Here, we present the details of the "evidence-on-the-evidence" which documents the impact of various biases on study outcomes. We also provide the details of the Cochrane findings on studies at uncertain risk of bias which we remarked upon in Part 1.

APPENDIX F: DELFINI SHORT CRITICAL APPRAISAL CHECKLIST—INTERVENTIONS FOR PREVENTION, SCREENING & THERAPY

We present here what we refer to as our "short" critical appraisal checklist. **Important**: This tool is in "shorthand," requiring understanding of the individual critical appraisal concepts listed or alluded to. We have already described other resources that you may find to help you further understand the details of critical appraisal, if you so desire. However, this list provides you with a roundup of the essential core concepts for critically appraising interventions for prevention, screening and therapy.

APPENDIX A: EBM TERMS FOR *EVERYONE*—A BRIEF ORIENTATION TO CRITICAL APPRAISAL

The following information may be of help in connecting with customers. Even though many customers will not be familiar with this information, you can use this information to help educate and establish common ground.

Critical Appraisal: A Short Description

As we have described, in the context of this book, **critical appraisal** means the evaluation of medical research for its likely **reliability** and its **clinical usefulness**. *All* studies and health information sources that reference studies should be critically appraised for **validity** and **clinical usefulness**.

While there are different approaches to evaluating a clinical trial for internal validity, good appraisers have in common a good understanding of bias and chance, knowing the potential for these study flaws to distort study results, and they share an understanding of what constitutes clinical usefulness. Our methods are consistent with those of many groups including The Cochrane Collaboration [Higgins 11] and the writers of the JAMA Users Guides to the Medical Literature [Guyatt 08]. Details of our work can be found on our website at www.delfini.org.

The process of critical appraisal entails reading a published study and looking for threats to reliability by examining all aspects of the study in an attempt to answer the question, "Does anything other than the intervention explain the results?"

Therefore, when it comes to medical science, we have **three essential questions**:

1. Is it true?

2. Is it useful?

3. Is it usable?

Critical appraisal is concerned with the first two of these questions. Effective critical appraisal is a combination of understanding critical appraisal concepts and applying clinical knowledge and critical thinking to continually ask, "Could anything explain the reported study results other than truth?"—in the case of therapeutic interventions, "truth" meaning a cause and effect relationship between an intervention of interest and a clinical outcome. If we believe that the results are probably true, we are then concerned with whether or not they are clinically useful.

After a study is evaluated for validity and clinical usefulness, then the study may be evaluated for "external validity" which is the "truth" of the study outside of the context of the study. Assessing external validity is often a matter of judgment based on looking at the contextual issues of the research and trying to gauge likely fit such as evaluating the reproducibility of the context for care, assessing comparability in compliance, comparing the characteristics of studied patients to a population for care or to an individual patient, etc.

Medical Research Study Types

At its most basic level, study designs are either **observational** or they are **experiments**.

Observations
In observations, you observe what happens naturally. We will have much more to say about observational studies later in the book when we talk about **"real world data"** in **Appendix B**.

Experiments
In an experiment, the patient is assigned an intervention, resulting in a situation in which neither the patient nor the patient's physician selects his or her intervention. **If choice is involved, the research is observational.**

Primary Studies
"Primary studies" refers to publications of the original research.

Secondary Studies
Sometimes researchers perform a collective analysis of multiple studies together and report on their findings. Such a review is called a **secondary study** (a meta-analysis is a type of secondary study) and ideally is undertaken in a formal way, which is called a **"systematic review."** Here are some key points about secondary studies—

- To perform a secondary study, researchers gather and analyze results of more than one study.

- "Systematic reviews" are secondary studies which are developed in a formal way based on generally agreed-upon industry standards with processes for posing clinical questions, searching and applying criteria for inclusion and quality.

- Systematic reviews should be evaluated at two levels—the quality of the science included in the review and the quality of the review itself.

- When high quality systematic reviews include reliable studies, they appear to be as reliable as high quality RCTs.

- However, because they involve multiple studies, critical appraisal of systematic reviews is more complex than evaluating a single RCT.

- "Narrative reviews," also known as "overviews," use informal methods for summarizing results from more than one study and frequently do not employ formal methods for searching, validity assessments or statistical assessments, among other procedures and, therefore, are potentially prone to the biases of the authors. Narrative reviews can be useful for background information or to learn about care options—but because of bias, generally they should not be used to inform medical decision-making.

- Unfortunately, many systematic reviews are also highly prone to bias frequently because of inattention to the quality of primary studies used in the secondary study —we have found this to be true in our experience, and this is documented in findings published by others, [Brok 08, Egger 03, Hennekens 12-09; Hennekens 04-09, Le Lorier 97].

Secondary Sources

By **secondary sources,** we mean medical information sources that utilize primary and secondary studies. Frequently secondary sources rely heavily on expert opinion and may contain both high and low quality evidence. Examples of secondary sources include clinical guidelines and recommendations, health care economic studies, disease management protocols, etc.

Unfortunately, we and others find that many secondary sources are also highly prone to bias, again frequently because of inattention to the quality of primary studies used in the secondary source [AHRQ 09, Grilli 00, Giannakakis 02, Jefferson 02, Stone 05].

Bias, Confounding and Chance—or Causality: The Four Explanations for Outcomes

There are **four possible explanations for the relationship**—or the association—between study interventions and study outcomes: bias, confounding (a special form of bias), chance or causality (truth). So to express this in another brief way, we can say that research results can be explained by bias, chance or truth. If we know that the likelihood of bias and chance is low, we can then accept the results as "likely to be true."

Bias

Bias is something that **"systematically" leads away from truth**—which simply means that something in the study—for example, lack of blinding—is leading the results away from the truth ("systematically" simply meaning something not due to random chance).

Confounding

Confounding is a special form of bias in which we think something has caused an outcome, but it is something else—hence we are "confounded" or confused by the confounder. A classic example is research reporting that taking vitamins reduces the risk of coronary heart disease when, in fact, people who take vitamins are more likely to do other things that reduce their risk. So in this instance, studies reporting lower cardiovascular event rates in patients taking vitamins were confounded by the "healthy user" effect.

Chance

A chance effect is just that—it is a **random accident**.

Cause and effect: truth.

A major goal of critical appraisal is to uncover bias, confounding and chance effects that may distort the reported study results. If we can **rule out** these potential explanations for the reported study results, we can then conclude that the results are likely to be because of causality—meaning that the results are likely to be due to the intervention being studied. For this reason, critical appraisal largely focuses on study problems, not on positive aspects of studies.

When it comes to medical interventions, **causality is the name of the game**. "If I take this pill, or if I have this intervention, what will happen to me?" Or the flip side, which is, "I got better. Am I better *because* of the intervention or because of some other reason?" Or "Do I only think I am better, but I really am not."

The second key question is one of **probability**—what is the likelihood of an outcome happening to me, either good or bad? Medications and other interventions don't always work the same for everyone. And so we look to medical science to help answer who is likely to benefit and who is likely to experience a harm. We look at the number of events that occurred in each study group and compare how many people benefited or were harmed.

This often gets distilled into a measure of outcome called "number-needed-to-treat" or the NNT, which answers the question, "How many patients need to be treated with this intervention, and within what time period, to benefit one person as compared to the other intervention studied?"

The complement of the number-needed-to-treat is the number-needed-to-harm—or the NNH—which is a measure of how many people need to be treated for one person to experience a harm who would not have experienced a harm if receiving the other intervention that was studied.

Also, sometimes good study design cannot be followed. It would be unethical to randomize patients to smoke cigarettes or not, for example, and it is sometimes impossible to blind a treatment. A critical appraiser cannot "forgive" these impossibilities because reality does not make an "allowance" for difficulty, and it is not the efforts of the researchers that are being evaluated or graded, but how confident we are in the study findings.

To determine cause and effect, we need to isolate the potential cause. To do so, we need groups to compare that are identical and treated exactly the same except for the one thing we are studying. We then **look at the results to see if the groups differed in outcomes**.

Remember that bias is anything that systematically leads away from truth. **Any difference** between groups other than what is being studied is automatically a bias because that difference could explain or distort study results.

Again, effective critical appraisal is a combination of understanding critical appraisal concepts and applying clinical knowledge and critical thinking to continually ask, **"Could anything explain the reported study results other than cause and effect?"**

Clinical Usefulness

Clinical usefulness—or meaningful clinical benefit—concerns whether the reported **results are big enough to benefit patients in clinically meaningful ways**. An **outcome**—also referred to as an "endpoint"—is what we are interested in studying. Typically these are **events** that patients experience such as pain or mortality, and studies may focus on reduction in events such as "reduction in mortality" or they may focus on improvements such as in "improved quality of life." Research that benefits patients in clinically meaningful ways addresses 5 key areas—and these are important to always keep in mind: 1) **morbidity**; 2)

mortality; 3) **symptom relief**; 4) mental, physical and emotional **functioning**; and, 5) health-related **quality of life.**

If an endpoint does not fall into one of these 5 topic areas, then it is called an **intermediate outcome marker**, some synonyms for which include "intermediate markers," "proxy markers," "surrogate markers" and "surrogate endpoints." An intermediate marker represents an outcome that is not directly experienced by people such as a biomarker or a lab or imaging test outcome (e.g., blood pressure measurement, hemoglobin A1c test or x-ray, etc.) Intermediate markers are outcome measures that are "assumed" to represent clinical outcomes (i.e., one of the 5 key areas listed above). As an example, "*blood pressure*" is often used as a surrogate endpoint in studies of stroke when the clinically significant outcome we are actually hoping to achieve is "*reduction in stroke*," which falls into the clinically significant categories of morbidity and mortality. But intermediate markers may or may not truly predict a clinically useful outcome. Effective critical appraisal requires a direct causal chain of proof of meaningful clinical benefit to accept the value of an intermediate marker.

Meaningful clinical benefit is a judgment based on the outcome and the size of the difference between groups reported in a valid study.

The 4 Stages of a Clinical Trial

There are four stages of a clinical trial that are evaluated for potential bias or chance effects and which we use as a framework for our critical appraisal work.

Selection & Treatment Assignment
Some important considerations include who was studied, how were they selected for study, are there enough people, how were they assigned to their study groups, and are the groups balanced?

Study Performance: Intervention & Context
What is being studied, and what is it being compared to? What else happened to study subjects in the course of the study?

Data Collection & Loss of Data
What information was collected, and how was it collected? What data are missing, and do missing data meaningfully distort the study results? A consideration includes whether results are distorted by lack of information due to missing patients or patients who are unable to complete their course of treatment.

Results & Assessing the Differences in the Outcomes of the Study Groups

How are differences in outcomes between the groups evaluated? What are those differences, and what is their potential meaning?

Critical Appraisal: A Sample of What One Looks Like

The case below is a fictional one. We present first the study abstract from a hypothetical journal, followed by our critical appraisal in which we list the hypothetical threats to validity in this made-up study.

Important: In looking at this example, keep in mind that we have only presented an abstract here. Abstracts can sometimes be useful by themselves to determine if a study is worth evaluating. However, abstracts are insufficient for determining that a study is valid. In this case, we are not showing you the "full published study." This example is to show you what a critical appraisal may look like.

DELFINI CRITICAL APPRAISAL CASE STUDY

HYPOTHETICAL CASE STUDY

MYOCEPTIMAB PREVENTS CARDIOVASCULAR MORBIDITY

Critical Appraisers & Date: Sheri A. Strite & Michael E. Stuart MD, Delfini Group; April Fool's Day, Any Year

PUBLISHED ABSTRACT

Background

Elevated myoreactive protein has been demonstrated to be associated with increased risk of myocardial infarction (MI). Myoceptimab is an inhibitor of myoreactive protein and has been shown to reduce myoreactive protein levels.

Methods

We conducted a randomized, double-blind trial in the Beaverton University Heart Care Center to assess the efficacy and safety in patients ages 55 and older who were at increased risk for cardiovascular events and had elevated myoreactive protein levels above 4 mg/L on two separate occasions. Patients were randomly assigned to receive 60 mg of myoceptimab (29 patients) or placebo (35 patients) daily for 6 months.

The study outcome was cardiovascular morbidity as defined by mean reduction of elevated levels of myoreactive protein, onset of new angina, admission to the hospital for any cardiovascular-related condition, myocardial infarction, stroke, claudication, heart failure or cardiovascular death.

Results

At 6 months, active treatment resulted in significantly reduced mean levels of myoreactive protein by 37%, reduced cardiovascular morbidity (n = 19 [65.5%] vs. n = 7 [20%]; P = 0.0003), and significantly more patients had a >50% increase in quality of life. There were no reported differences in safety outcomes.

Conclusions

Treatment with myoceptimab reduced cardiovascular morbidity and was associated with significant beneficial effects on quality of life. Myoceptimab offers a safe and effective therapeutic option for patients who are at increased risk for cardiovascular events.

DELFINI CRITICAL APPRAISAL

- Study size: small
- Primary endpoint: questionable composite
- Randomization: not truly randomized; patients assigned to groups by study consent date
- Concealment of allocation: no details
- Baseline characteristics: slightly higher rate of angina in the placebo group
- Blinding: insufficient details and no indication of blind assessment
- Intergroup differences: participating cardiologists were not restricted in patient management so as to replicate real-world conditions; no details of co-interventions reported between groups
- Attrition: less than 1 percent
- Safety, including long term harms, is uncertain
- Results assessment: questionable clinical significance, selective reporting and *post-hoc* results
- Critical appraisal conclusion: uncertain validity

Another example of a critical appraisal is available here at our website: http://www.delfini.org/delfiniClick_QI.htm#delfinicriticalappraisal_gerd

PICOTS

A useful framework for an external validity assessment, among other things, is PICOTS which stands for patient, intervention, comparator, outcome, timing and setting [Atkins 08]. We actually add an additional dimension—**PICPOTS**—the second "P" standing for performance issues, which would include such things as care experiences other than the intervention such as co-interventions, adherence, etc. This is also a useful list when considering heterogeneity between studies.

Evidence Grading

Once a study has been critically appraised, many evaluators assign a grade. Usually an evidence grade is a summary expression of the quality and/or the clinical usability of the evidence. The grade itself may be applied to the overall study or to a study element such as a reported result or to an assessment of the overall strength of the evidence when considering a combination of studies—for example, a secondary study such as a meta-analysis.

There are many different grading systems currently in use, so to understand the meaning behind the grade, you need to look up the criteria for the system and be aware that a grade of Level 1 evidence in one system, for example, might have a different meaning than Level 1 in another system. Also, criteria may be problematic, allowing low quality studies to receive a high grade.

For more information on critical appraisal, visit our website at www.delfini.org.

APPENDICES FOR OUR PRESCRIPTION: A MAP OF THE 5 MILESTONES LEADING TO EFFECTIVE EVIDENCE COMMUNICATION WITH CUSTOMERS—RRAPP™

APPENDIX B: DETAILS FOR "RESEARCH ~ High Quality & Clinically Useful Evidence"

Conduct high-quality research on appropriate populations using good comparators and selecting useful endpoints that are meaningful to customers. Strive for solid research design and good execution, working to maximize good study performance outcomes and utilizing effective measurement methods.

The selected study design and performance elements that we expound upon in this appendix are these—

- Appropriate populations for study;

- Comparators;

- Endpoints generally and endpoints and other considerations for oncology studies;

- Maximizing good study performance outcomes (e.g., successful blinding is an example of a "study performance outcome");

- Effective measurement methods; and,

- "Real world data" and CER (comparative effectiveness research).

We also address research issues for **diagnostic testing** and **screening**. However, because these two areas have many complexities and special considerations, we are not addressing them in this section, but rather we depart from our categories and discuss both research issues and reporting ideals together for greater clarity and simplicity in **Appendix C: Reporting.**

Important: **If you are interested in trial design**, note that there will be other pieces of information that may be very useful to you in **subsequent appendices**. For example, in **Appendix D: Details For "Prepare To Connect Over The Evidence ~ Know The Customer to Interact with the Customer,"** we discuss some data imputation methods, including problems with "last observation carried forward" (LOCF). In that section, our purpose is to address what customers may or may not know to evaluate. However, that discussion—and other discussions in other appendices regardless of their title—may be of value to you. So we encourage reading through all the information we have provided for you in this book.

As you read these items, keep in mind that sometimes customer desires are going to be in conflict with research realities. Customer staff, even if skilled critical appraisers, are unlikely to have experience as research trialists and so, at times, they may express puzzlement or frustration that populations for study are sicker or healthier than those in the customer's population, to use one example. Bear in mind that customers are end users of research results and that this is what drives their needs and wants from research.

Appropriate Populations

One of the chief concerns of customers is that subjects studied are frequently not perceived to be similar to the populations for which these customers are responsible. The issue is whether study results are likely to be realized outside of the study population, i.e., in the customer's population. We've talked some about internal validity which is the truth of the study within its own context. We are now stepping outside of that into the truth of the study *outside* of its study context—this is referred to as "external validity."

Considerations include how similar real-world patients are to studied populations and the ability to successfully apply the intervention that was studied and replicate other circumstances of care or other conditions that could affect the outcomes experienced by patients. As an example, customers have concerns whether adherence in practice will be similar to that in trials—and in all likelihood, it is doubtful that it will be. Also, if only young and healthy people or people without comorbidities are studied, it's very reasonable to expect that study results will not be likely to be replicated in practice. Therefore, a typical observation made by customers is that their patients are sicker, healthier or in some other way different from the population studied.

Another typical comment that we hear from customers is that the study population is very heterogeneous. This may encourage the greater use of analysis of subpopulations. However, any such subgroups should be prespecified (also referred to as *a priori*) to reduce the likelihood of "finding" statistically significant differences that, in truth, are really due to chance. Subgroup analyses that are not prespecified should only be considered hypothesis-generating, which may also be true even for prespecified analyses if many are done because of the increased potential for chance effects. We would also recommend that any such analyses include a caution about the potential of non-significant findings to be the result of insufficient power (not enough people) and not truly reflective of no difference between the groups—an area that many customers misunderstand.

There can be other ways in which populations can be problematic. There are ways in which subjects may be recruited which could affect outcomes. For example, assume we are planning to conduct a trial of drug A for alcohol dependence. The baseline characteristics of study subjects are likely to differ significantly if subjects are enrolled from inpatient alcohol treatment facilities rather than enrolling subjects who respond to print media or live media requests for enrollment. Outcomes may differ between the two groups because of numerous differences in health status and demographic variables (e.g., those enrolled from inpatient centers are likely to be much sicker). Another example: if patients who have been misdiagnosed are enrolled in a trial, that will clearly have implications for study results. If a patient is familiar with side effects of the treatment to which he or she has been assigned, that could bias the study by unblinding the patient and his or her care providers. If patients who have failed the treatment are subsequently enrolled in a study assessing that same treatment, the deck will be stacked in favor of the comparison treatment. Upon reading, these may seem obvious; however, we see problems like these in clinical trials all the time.

Comparators

Often customers express frustration when studies utilize a placebo comparator. Because making indirect comparisons between studies can be unreliable, customers cry out for head-to-head trials. In fact, many customers miss the importance of having a placebo comparator. We think head-to-head trials are great, but we advocate the inclusion of a placebo arm whenever ethically possible.

A controversy was created in the VIGOR trial due to the absence of a placebo comparison group. The VIGOR (Vioxx GI Outcomes Research) study was a clinical trial comparing the upper gastrointestinal toxicity of the COX-2 inhibitor, rofecoxib (trade name Vioxx), versus naproxen, an over-the-counter anti-inflammatory drug used for arthritis and pain in the same family as aspirin and ibuprofen [Bombardier 00]. The published study reported some very concerning safety data showing a difference in myocardial infarction between groups. The authors concluded, "[Our] results are consistent with the theory that naproxen has a coronary protective effect and highlight the fact that rofecoxib does not provide this type of protection owing to its selective inhibition of cyclooxygenase-2 at its therapeutic doses and at higher doses." While naproxen would be a better treatment choice given the benefit-to-harm ratio, a placebo comparison group would have made it clear that the outcomes were due to safety issues with Vioxx.

Another problem with the lack of placebo comparator can arise in a head-to-head trial if the active agents do not already have studies that prove their efficacy. Remember that most of the studies evaluated by skilled evaluators fail a rigorous critical appraisal. Therefore, there is a reasonable possibility that a head-to-head trial without a placebo comparator—particularly using a non-inferiority or equivalence design—could be comparing two ineffective agents or two agents whose efficacy is uncertain.

When designing head-to-head trials, researchers should be scrupulous about giving the comparator a fair shake. Some studies utilize suboptimal dosing for the comparator, for example. Many customers miss a lot when it comes to identifying bias in studies; however, customers tend to be very aware of dosing differences. Frequently when investigators choose a poor comparator, they provide lengthy explanations for their choice. Customers frequently view these explanations as window dressing and become mistrustful—a situation that helps nobody.

Endpoints

First, we want to remind you of the five meaningful outcomes that benefit patients: 1) morbidity; 2) mortality; 3) symptom relief; 4) functioning; and, 5) quality of life. Any other outcome is an intermediate marker and requires a causal "proof of evidence" chain.

One of the biggest concerns that we hear from customers is that they are often unhappy with endpoints reported in industry-sponsored research. This tends to happen if the endpoint is one that does not appear to be of meaningful clinical benefit. What customers may not always appreciate is that sometimes these endpoints are dictated by the FDA. However, regardless of FDA requirements or input, chosen endpoints for study need to be perceived as providing meaningful clinical benefit to patients. Customers are looking for value, and most interventions pose risk of harm. Therefore, we advise that you work with customers or others who can advise you on meaningful clinical benefit at the outset of the design of the study to ensure that outcomes of interest to customers get included in the study along with those required by the FDA.

Investigators are also well-advised to be careful when selecting outcomes for combining into composite endpoints. Good composite endpoints are valid, reasonable, fair and clinically useful. Customers are alert to notice endpoints in a combination which are likely to inadvertently or unfairly drive the outcomes or which are under the control of one of the investigators or someone else participating in the research ("admission to the hospital" is an example of an endpoint that is subject to the control of someone involved in the research). In short, customers look for whether or not there is any way that the construction of the combined endpoint is likely to favor the intervention. Some areas to which reviewers pay close attention include—

1. Subjective outcomes especially if no blinding;

2. Combinations including severe outcomes with mild ones, process measures, intermediate markers without a direct chain of causality to a clinical outcome and, as we mentioned, items under control or influence of a participant in the research;

3. Potential for double-counting;

4. If applicable, inclusion of all relevant events;

5. How meaningfully-related the combination is;

6. Whether there are other ways the combination could be misleading (e.g., disease-free survival when a treatment reduces risk of tumor recurrence, but increases risk of death); and,

7. Whether researchers reported results on the individual components or not. Without this information, depending upon the combination, a situation could result in which symptoms decreased, but mortality increased, but the composite masks this untoward outcome (e.g., as in the example above).

Composite endpoints are frequently developed for efficacy because of increased power to show a difference between groups, but composites are rarely used for safety. More sophisticated reviewers may be alert to this and know that individual safety outcomes are less likely to differ between groups than if combined and that reporting only individual safety outcome differences "allows" investigators to conclude that there was no difference in adverse event rates between the groups.

Also, be aware that some customers are automatically dismissive of secondary outcomes generally and that many will reject statistically significant secondary outcomes if the primary outcome has not achieved significance. If we were designing a study, we would keep this in mind and be careful to establish meaningful primary outcomes for which statistical significance is likely to be reachable.

Endpoints and Other Considerations for Oncology Studies

Oncology studies pose special challenges. Often, the trials have small populations and are of short duration. Frequently, questions are raised about the clinical meaningfulness of differences between groups such as overall survival, even when statistically significant, when the differences are very small such as a few weeks increased survival. Further, what a small difference actually means may be obscured by the results reporting. When means are reported, do the results represent a few people doing very well for a long period of time or are they reflective instead of many people in the study group experiencing a short term benefit. This becomes important when considering a possibility of a very meaningful benefit in a subgroup of patients more likely to be responsive to a treatment as compared to a majority of patients reported as experiencing a small benefit.

An important issue is what kind of endpoint is used. The use of surrogate outcome measures is common, and tumor response assessments which are frequently used, may not be a good proxy for survival. Reductions in tumor size following therapy do not always represent an improvement in the prognosis, and for this reason, overall survival is the ideal measurement in oncology trials. However, various tumor assessments are frequently employed as primary or secondary endpoints in oncology studies. Historically, adequacy of tumor treatments has been measured by assessing tumor recurrence, disappearance, time-to-progression of tumors, the appearance of new tumors and measurements of tumor size. In some studies, these measurements are carried out at various anatomical sites, and the totals are summed. Various imaging modalities are utilized in assessing tumors. Bias can occur when there are errors in any of these measurements.

In oncology research, from a critical appraisal standpoint, the outcome of mortality is highly clinically significant. "**Overall survival**" is the preferred primary outcome and is defined as the time from randomization until death from any cause and is measured in the intent-to-treat population (i.e., all randomized subjects analyzed by their assigned group).

Next ranking in endpoint quality are composite endpoints that include mortality— depending, of course, on the appropriateness of the individual endpoints.

Also, quality of life and functioning may be important endpoints to study in the absence of true survival information.

Other endpoints used in oncology studies are these, each of which is prone to tumor assessment bias:

- **Progression-free Survival** (PFS) is generally defined as the time from randomization until objective tumor progression or death. This outcome has been used by the FDA for some accelerated approvals.

- **Disease-free Survival**, which is defined as the time from randomization until recurrence of tumor or death from any cause.

- **Objective Response Rate**, which is defined as the proportion of patients with tumor size reduction of a predefined amount and for a minimum time period.

- **Time-to-Progression**, which is defined as the time from randomization until objective tumor progression.

Time-to-Treatment Failure is defined as a composite endpoint measuring time from randomization to discontinuation of treatment for any reason, including disease progression, treatment toxicity and death. It is not recommended as a regulatory approval endpoint because it is likely to report biased outcomes as it does not adequately distinguish efficacy from other variables.

In general, another important critical appraisal consideration is that, if patients' outcomes are measured until tumor progression and are still followed until death, there is potential for confounding of results post-progression if another treatment is utilized and the studied groups are not balanced in these subsequent treatments.

Maximize Good Study Performance Outcomes

Study quality is determined by quality in study design, methodology, execution and "study performance outcomes." By good "study performance outcomes," we mean how well a study performance area has met with success. One example is the likely success of blinding. It's one thing to design good blinding methods and implement them. It's another thing entirely for blinding to have been effectively achieved. And so *success of blinding* is a *study performance outcome*.

Other examples of study performance outcomes are adequacy of the randomization process which includes generation of the randomization sequence and success of concealment of allocation to study groups, quality control checks with resulting successes, protocol compliance, adherence, completeness and correctness of data capture, retention of balance between groups and low attrition (although, the attrition area is more complex in that attrition may or may not result in attrition bias, not counting issues resulting from smaller sample sizes).

We will use blinding for further illustration. One of the few areas that we are going to specifically address in this section is how to give blinding a chance of success using one of the most neglected key study elements and that is concealment of allocation to study groups. We will also make a short comment about a selected protocol compliance issue—and that is early stopping of clinical trials, especially for benefit.

Blinding

In our opinion, blinding is one of the most important critical appraisal considerations. Researchers have reported that lack of blinding is likely to overestimate benefit by up to a relative 72% [Juni 01, Kjaergard 01, Poolman 07, Schulz 95]. Ultimately requirements for successful blinding include no one knowing the study group to which a patient is assigned and no one knowing the study intervention a patient receives (e.g., a patient might be treated by care providers differently because of "knowledge" of group assignment, but inadvertently have gotten the wrong treatment and so both considerations are important in successful blinding). When we evaluate blinding, we are looking at several things. Was the way in which patients were assigned to their study group hidden so that no one could affect group assignment? This is referred to as "concealment of allocation." Were the interventions disguised so that they could not be distinguished? Were there any differences in the performance of the study that could unblind patient treatment assignment? For example, if a chemotherapeutic agent with a high-frequency of alopecia (hair loss) as a side effect was compared to placebo, the study could not be considered to be successfully blinded. Were assessors blinded?

In our estimation, blinding is so important that we would expect that evidence-savvy groups would be very attuned to the need for successful blinding. Some reviewers believe that blinding only matters in the case of subjective outcomes such as pain. Certainly, there can be great opportunity for bias in such instances. If I know that I'm getting an active agent, I may be more likely to believe and report that I'm experiencing pain relief than if I know I'm receiving placebo. Or if my clinician knows that I am receiving an active agent, he or she may be very encouraging and relate to me differently in some way that makes me feel better or that results in my reporting a better outcome.

However, blinding is important in objective outcomes as well—even a "hard outcome" such as death. Clinicians certainly can impact patient mortality. (In our training programs, if someone suggests that blinding only matters for subjective outcomes, we sometimes respond back by posing this as a question to the physicians in the room to make our point. "Do you think you can affect the life of a patient?" we ask. They all nod back enthusiastically.) If the study is not successfully blinded, it is possible that a clinician's care choices may be affected by knowledge of an intervention, and these choices could affect the life of a patient.

The RECORD trial is instructive of the importance of blinding even in the presence of objective outcomes. The RECORD trial (Rosiglitazone Evaluated for Cardiac Outcomes and Regulation of Glycemia in Diabetes) is an example of an open-label (i.e., unblinded) trial in which lack of blinding, except for assessors, led to a suspected biased mortality assessment that appears to have significantly altered results. Prespecified safety outcomes included drug-related mortality which was initially determined by patients' unblinded physicians and then confirmed or rejected by blinded adjudicators. It was determined that event rates for myocardial infarction (MI) in the control group were unexpectedly low, which led to an independent review by the FDA which identified myriad problems with case report forms created prior to any blind assessment [Psaty 10]. The FDA review resulted in a re-analysis [Marciniak 10], using the available readjudicated case information with the end result that the outcome of non-significance for risk of MI in the original study report changed to a statistically significant difference, the results of which were "remarkably close" to results reported in the original meta-analysis that raised concerns about rosiglitazone and cardiovascular risk in the first place [Nissen 07].

As we've stated before, attrition is not necessarily the same as attrition bias, not counting issues associated with smaller sample size. We make mention of it here, however, because lack of effective blinding can result in attrition bias. Let's imagine a study in which patients are on an active agent or placebo. And now let us imagine that care was not taken to conceal assignment of patients to their study groups. A physician who knows his or her patient is on placebo might be more likely to be impatient about treatment outcomes and encourage a patient to seek other treatment as compared to a physician who knows his or her patient is receiving the active agent. Therefore, the resulting attrition would be due to bias and, in this example, the results may be meaningfully distorted if a sufficient number of physicians acted in this manner and their patients complied.

Every attempt should be made to successfully blind a study. There are instances in which people claim studies cannot be blinded, such as in cases of surgical interventions. However, investigators should make significant efforts to successfully blind all individuals involved in studies and who work with study data because knowledge of treatment assignment can significantly affect results. When blinding is difficult or not possible, some people have a tendency to try and "forgive" the researchers. But validity is about reliability of results, not researcher challenges and efforts—validity isn't something that can "bend" to provide allowance for difficulty. Therefore, it is important to do everything possible to maximize any potential blinding and seek ways to mitigate the potential compromise of group assignment and the effects of treatment knowledge.

Success of Concealed Allocation: A Requirement for the Likely Success of Blinding

Concealment of allocation means concealing the study group assignments in such a way that nobody can affect an individual patient's assignment to his or her designated study group. Effective blinding starts with randomization because it is unpredictable. Following generation of the randomization sequence, concealment of allocation (again, hiding the assignment to study group) is the next step leading to the potential for successful blinding. Unfortunately, it is rarely addressed in study protocols or—more importantly, in publications or post-study supplementary information. And yet, it is one of the most important of study elements.

The CAPPP Trial [Hansson 99] is instructive of what appears to be a failure to conceal allocation of subjects to their groups as there is good evidence that study assignment was manipulated. The goal of this trial was to compare captopril, an ACE inhibitor (angiotensin-converting enzyme inhibitor), and what at that time was considered to be conventional therapy— diuretics and beta-blockers. Outcomes included cardiovascular morbidity (e.g., fatal and non-fatal stroke) and mortality in patients with hypertension.

At the conclusion of the trial, the results surprisingly showed an increase in a combined outcome of fatal and non-fatal stroke in the captopril group—a very unexpected outcome. Subsequently, a prominent biostatistician analyzed the baseline characteristics and reported in a letter to the editor that the small, but highly significant differences, between the two treatment groups in several baseline characteristics—height, weight, systolic and diastolic blood pressure (with respective p-values of 10 to the minus 4th power, 10 to the minus 3rd power, 10 to the minus 8th power, and 10 to the minus 18th power

"...show that the process of randomisation by sealed numbered envelopes was frequently violated. Presumably, at some centres those responsible for entering patients sometimes unsealed the envelopes before the next patient was formally entered, and then let knowledge of what the next treatment would be influence their decision as to whether that patient should be entered and assigned that foreknown treatment [Peto 99]." In other words, the likely unblinding of the study for some patients at the point at which those patients were allocated to their study groups created significant bias that seriously compromised the study results.

In all likelihood, this happened because of the desire of individual physicians to give their patients the "latest" and "best" opportunity for good outcomes such as lower blood pressure and risk of stroke. What appears likely is that physicians manipulated study assignment for their patients at greater risk. This, then, is the likely cause of the prognostic risk imbalance between the study groups that resulted in biased results indicating that captopril may cause stroke, when, in fact, difference in stroke rates could have been due to flawed concealment of allocation through use of envelopes.

It would seem that having to protect study group assignment from manipulation would only matter in rare occasions. However, you never know what might drive such behavior in humans. This area has been considered to be so important that The Cochrane Collaboration in the past has called this out as a key study quality indicator.

Sheri was discussing concealment of allocation with a colleague on one occasion. With some embarrassment, he confessed to her that he was aware of an instance in which medical residents were to enroll consenting patients in a clinical trial using a box of envelopes that contained a code to assign patients to their study groups. Assignment to the intervention group required an additional workup (a problem in and of itself in that there should be no differences between care experiences in the groups except for the intervention being studied).

Residents were supervised on the day shift; however, they were not supervised at night. On the night shift, at the point of assigning a patient to his or her group, frequently the resident would hold the envelope up to the light, and if the assignment was to the intervention group, to the back of the box that envelope would go. As you can imagine, patients that come in for care during the daytime where care is likely to be scheduled and orderly may be very different from those patients that present for care in the middle of the night, potentially resulting in very different groups. And if groups differ, study outcomes might be a result of those differences and not the intervention under study. In this case, we would likely have a sicker population in the comparison group and a healthier population in the intervention group—the result of which would give an advantage to the intervention.

We also know of another instance in which a study was compromised due to intentional human behavior. While this following example is not about concealment of allocation, it is further support that humans may manipulate study activities in their own interest or in their perceived best interest for their patients, which is assumably what happened in the CAPPP Trial. In this example, a growth hormone agent was being compared to placebo. Both agents were administered intravenously. One of the hospital staff was convinced that the growth hormone would improve outcomes for patients and that it was unethical not to provide this agent to all infants who had been enrolled in the study. Therefore, this individual managed to achieve administration of the active agent to all patients. (In fact, the reason the agent was being studied was to *learn* whether it worked or not.) Because research is about looking at the difference in outcomes between groups, by ensuring that all patients, regardless of study group assignment, received the active agent, the staffer engineered an outcome in which there would be no difference between the groups—exactly the opposite of what she was hoping for and believing. Fortunately, this was a multi-center trial.

Examples of appropriate methods to conceal allocation include the use of centralized call centers, computerized interactive voice response systems (IVRS) and identical locked containers to hide the allocation code which are in control of someone not otherwise involved in the study. Sometimes you will see that opaque envelopes are used; however, envelopes can be easily manipulated—so we would look for additional protections before accepting this method even though The Cochrane Collaboration, at the time of this writing, approves of this technique. Customers that we train are alert to this.

Early Stopping for Benefit

For our last example of issues in study performance we will briefly mention early stopping of trials for benefit—a problem we are seeing with increasing frequency. The issue is trials being stopped early because a statistically significant difference between outcomes has been identified during an interim analysis. Sophisticated reviewers are aware that the early stopping of the trial for efficacy at a stage in the trial where very few outcome events have occurred may result in a high likelihood of chance outcomes [Bassler 10, Guyatt 12].

And so, to recap, in this section we have just given you some information on concealment of allocation and early stopping for benefit as examples of study performance outcomes. Again, other examples of study performance outcomes are adequacy of the randomization process which includes generation of the randomization sequence, quality control checks with resulting successes, protocol compliance, adherence, completeness and correctness of data capture, retention of balance between groups and, ideally, low attrition.

Effective Measurement Methods

Some customers will be very alert to when a nonstandard instrument or method is chosen for measurement. As we point out to learners in our critical appraisal workshops, it doesn't take much to earn the label "validated," and often validation criteria are largely, if not fully, subject to judgment. We've seen instances in which industry has created a measurement tool which has given their intervention some advantage. When this happens and if critical appraisers discover it, trust becomes eroded, and everything gets harder for everyone—and ultimately patients suffer.

Another caution that we would give is to be very thoughtful about establishing your criteria for what equals response, improvement, etc. This is another area that customers do not tend to miss and are often unforgiving when they perceive that definitions for outcomes give an advantage to an intervention under investigation. For example, we have seen an instance in which a pain scale of over 100 points was used and in which a change of 3 points or more was defined as "improvement." The committee that reviewed this chucked the study (after rolling their eyes), and trust in the company became seriously challenged.

"Real World Data"

In recent years, attention has been focused increasingly on **comparative effectiveness research (CER)** and "**real world data**." Customers want comparisons of various drugs or interventions, they want those comparisons under "real world" conditions, and they want answers fast. Customers also often have access to a wealth of data. This combination of "wants" and the availability of organizational data can result in some very misleading "answers." Because of this increasing focus and its attendant risks, we will discuss this type of research at some length.

The first step in assessing the validity of a study is to match the study design to the clinical question. **To prove the efficacy of an intervention, the appropriate study design is an experiment.** At its most basic level, study designs are either observational or they are experiments. In observational studies, you observe what happens naturally. Observations can be useful to answer certain questions, but they are highly prone to bias and can almost never be relied upon to answer questions about cause and effect. Valid RCTs are required to reliably answer questions about cause and effect relationships with therapeutic interventions.

One reason for this is that there is a lack of equality in many "prognostic factors" between groups in observational studies. This lack of equality starts with how dissimilar the groups are to each other at the start. Furthermore, this is a problem that cannot be sufficiently addressed through statistical adjusting because many differences (confounders) are unknown and, therefore, cannot be adjusted. This lack of equality between groups in observational studies extends even deeper to such areas as differences in care such as differing co-interventions or other care experiences, measurement methods, length of time followed and more.

Another reason why observations can be misleading is that, generally, what is observed is a result of **choice**. Think back to our vitamin example in our definition of confounding in **Appendix A**. Those who choose to take vitamins are likely to choose to make many other healthy lifestyle-related choices which could actually be responsible for the reported research results.

Experiments take choice out of the equation by **assigning** subjects to the intervention to be studied or the comparison group. In fact, that is a quick way to tell whether a study is an observation or an experiment. If a patient or his or her physician *chose* the intervention under study, the study is observational.

With rare exception, experiments are required for answering questions of cause and effect. Therefore, experiments are the best study type for researching efficacy of therapies, unless the observations resulted in highly dramatic before-and-after outcomes, referred to as "**all-or-none results**." This is a very rare occurrence. For example, before the intervention, everyone died and after application of the intervention, almost no one died. When all-or-none results occur in observational studies, they are generally considered reliable. But only well-designed and conducted experiments, with good study performance outcomes, are considered truly reliable to establish cause and effect.

If subjects are not assigned to their study groups through randomization or through a restricted randomization process called minimization, the experiment can be highly prone to bias because the groups of subjects are likely to be different from each other, and those differences could affect or explain the study results. Inadequate generation of the randomization sequence has been found to distort study results as high as a relative 75% [Juni 01, Kjaergard 01, Savovic 12, van Tulder 09].

Fighting to Convince Us

Years ago, occasionally during our workshops a rare participant would approach us and try to convince us that observations could be just as trustable as RCTs. We then developed a new strategy of letting him or her do a quick critical appraisal, comparing observational study elements to those of RCTs. We no longer have to fight this battle, and this kind of challenge is a thing of the past.

The exercise goes like this—

Review the elements of the two studies described below. Answer whether you would find each study *potentially* reliable and worth a closer look based on the following information:

Study 1 Elements

1. There are two concurrent groups for study.

2. Baseline characteristics are similar between groups.

3. No adjustment has been made for the baseline characteristics.

4. Computer-generated random number table determines the intervention.

5. No one knows who gets which treatment.

6. A formal treatment protocol is used.

7. There is uniformity in use of co-interventions, measurement methods and treatment duration.

Study 2 Elements

1. There are two concurrent groups for study.

2. Baseline characteristics vary between groups.

3. The baseline characteristics were statistically adjusted.

4. Patients' physicians determine the patient's intervention.

5. Everyone knows who gets which treatment.

6. There is no treatment protocol.

7. There is no uniformity in use of co-interventions, measurement methods or treatment duration.

Uniformly, we get agreement that Study 1 could potentially be so reliable that it could garner a Grade A. We also get agreement that Study 2 cannot be considered reliable. We ask people to tell us the design of the two studies. People can easily identify that Study 1 is an RCT and that Study 2 is an observation. We then point out that Study 2 is the *best* that an observation can be. People nod in understanding. What many people forget is that, for the most part, "real world data" come from observations.

The Positive Predictive Values of Various Study Types
In a paper entitled, "Why Most Published Research Findings are False," the renown clinical epidemiologist, John Ioannidis, reported his findings on the positive predictive value of various study types [Ioannidis 05]. His calculations are as follows:

1. Well-done RCT—0.85

2. Meta-analysis of well-done RCTs—0.85

3. Meta-analysis of small, inconclusive RCTs—0.41

4. Well-done epidemiological (observational) study—0.20

5. Epidemiologic study with threats to validity—0.12

6. Discovery-oriented exploratory research—0.0010

In other words, his data indicate that an observational study is right only about 20% of the time. A problem is how would you know which time? The answer is that you could only know which observational study was right if you had confirmation of the observational study outcomes from at least one, but preferably several, well-designed and conducted double-blind, randomized controlled trials. With rare exception, only valid experiments, such as valid RCTs, can answer cause-and-effect questions such as the efficacy of an intervention.

Misleading Real World Studies

Based on the findings of Ioannidis and others, it is important to remember that all administrative claims data, observational data recorded in medical records, surveys and observational studies are more likely than not to provide false information about the effectiveness of interventions [Deeks 03, Ioannidis 05]. Observational data can be very useful when assessing adherence to drugs, compliance with guidelines, identifying populations for further study, generating hypotheses, assessing current practice patterns including cost issues and identifying early safety signals. However, *buyer beware* when it comes to assessing cause and effect relationships using observational data. Several examples are provided below.

Example 1: Losartan and candesartan have both been shown in RCTs to reduce cardiovascular mortality in some populations. However, by 2007, no head-to-head clinical trials had been performed. In order to compare the efficacy of these two drugs, several investigators used observational data from hospital discharge summaries to compare mortality outcomes between losartan and candesartan [Eklind-Cervenka 11, Hudson 07]. The reported results indicated a significant survival advantage for candesartan. However, an observational study in 2012 that utilized individual subject data reported no survival advantage for candesartan [Svanstrom 12]. The reason for the conflicting findings of the studies is likely to be that the 2012 study was able to adjust the data for dosage, cardiovascular and other clinical co-morbidities and co-interventions. Unfortunately, no matter what statistical methods are used for adjusting differences in baseline variables, observational studies are unable to reliably remove potential selection, performance, measurement, attrition and other biases.

Example 2 (Hypothetical): A new glaucoma drug is marketed as having fewer pulmonary adverse events than older drugs. Clinicians prescribe the new drug to high-risk chronic obstructive pulmonary disease (COPD) patients, and one group decides to examine their administrative claims data to see the effect of the new drug on hospital admissions for COPD. The clinicians are surprised to see a higher admission rate for the new drug. What happened here? The answer is that clinicians put all of their high-risk COPD patients on the new drug, and when they compared hospital admissions to those patients treated with older drugs, the results reflected the problem of selection bias. The results were misleading because the comparison groups were very different in terms of their disease severity, and this is the explanation for the higher admission rate in patients receiving the new drug. The technical term for this problem is "confounding by indication."

Example 3 (Hypothetical): Claims data reveal higher risk of suicide with Prozac when compared with older antidepressants. Explanation: Clinicians kept stabilized patients on the older medication, but switched severely depressed patients to the newer drug, Prozac. Again, we see here the common problem of selection bias in comparisons done with observational data.

In well-designed clinical trials, randomization would have created two equal groups in each of these examples, and the selection bias seen with the real world data problems would not have occurred.

In their understandable clamor for much needed head-to-head comparisons, in their sense of urgency for speedy information, in their desires for real world answers—in their potential hope for your funding to mine their "wealth" of data—customers may come to you to partner on these kinds of studies. You risk supporting highly invalid findings that could result in incorrect conclusions that your product is not as effective as another agent or presents a safety risk. No one benefits from this, despite the hopes, needs and clamoring. We have three words for you, and they are the same words: educate, educate, educate.

APPENDIX C: DETAILS FOR "REPORT ~ Clarity & Transparency"

Provide transparent reporting that is meaningful to customers. Understand if there are any gaps between your research and its reporting and take steps to make needed information accessible.

Investigators should pay close attention to the background statement and report on key information that allows assessors to evaluate the trial for design issues and selection, performance, measurement, attrition and assessment biases and any other threats to validity including the likelihood of chance effects. Investigators should also include a statement of limitations. Authors' conclusions should be meticulous in not overstating clinical benefits or minimizing potential harms. When studies are reported well, often critical appraisal can be accomplished quickly—a situation that makes everyone happy and is in patients' best interests.

Our Reporting Ideals for Clinical Trials

We present our general ideals here in the framework of how we think of the stages of a clinical trial when we are assessing validity. **This list should not necessarily be regarded as complete**—we have favored inclusion of items that are frequently omitted or worth discussing. However, an omission of an item from this list does not mean that we and other reviewers are not interested in information about that element.

Again, **because many customers are *not* familiar with these ideas, we take a shift in perspective to say "we look for" instead of "customers look for..."**

And speaking of omissions, here is a reminder that when key information is omitted from the publication of a study, **that omission goes on our list of threats to validity because of our uncertainty about risk of bias and the potential for the distorting effect of the bias on the reported results**. Below is a common approach utilized by many critical appraisers.

Subject Selection

1. How were subjects selected for study?

2. Inclusion and exclusion criteria

3. Table of baseline characteristics

Readers examine the table of baseline characteristics to see if important prognostic variables are similar in each group. Again, the term "prognostic variables" refers to demographic and clinical factors (e.g., age, blood pressure, etc.) that are known or believed to influence a subject's likelihood of responding to an intervention. If patients are assigned to their study groups by random chance, then it is likely that both known and unknown prognostic variables will be equally distributed among study groups. If baseline characteristics are similar, this suggests that randomization was successful.

4. How were subjects assigned to their groups?

If techniques were used such as randomization or minimization, investigators need to **provide details**. It is not sufficient to simply say the study was a randomized trial or include the word "randomization" in the title. (Because nearly everything we say about randomized controlled trials can be said about trials using minimization—we will not refer to the method of minimization again, but we will simply refer to RCTs.) Frequently, this can be a very short description, such as, "A computer-generated schedule was utilized to randomize patients," or "A computer-generated list of random numbers was used to allocate patients to groups." Readers also need details such as blocking and stratification methods, if those were used.

5. Disclose methods for concealing allocation of patients to their study groups.

This is discussed in detail in **Appendix B**. This too can be a very short description. If we see that an interactive voice response system (IVRS) was utilized, for example, that's all we need to be satisfied that concealment of allocation was likely.

6. Make it easy to identify the number of patients in each study group.

Study Performance

1. Identify details about the intervention under study and its comparator.

Generally for pharmaceutical and biotech agents, this information is excellently represented. Where this information often falls short is for other kinds of interventions. Authors should provide as much detail as they can that would enable a clinician to replicate the intervention. Another problem area is when the comparator is "usual care."

Investigators should provide as much detail as possible about what constituted usual care.

Another key piece of advice is that if you are utilizing an intervention that is sufficiently new or unusual that it requires specialized training, be sure to report on training and quality control measures and performance outcomes of quality control.

2. What outcomes will be evaluated?

Label outcomes so that they are **tagged with meaningful designations** such as primary outcomes, secondary outcomes and exploratory outcomes, clearly identifying which of these have been prespecified.

If you are selecting **intermediate outcomes** for study, be sure to provide a valid chain of evidence "proof" that supports the clinical meaningfulness of the outcome.

For **composite outcomes**, please include results for each outcome as well as for the composite endpoint.

3. Blinding

Who was blinded, and how were they blinded? We like to see a specific mention made of **blinded assessment** or a statement that all subjects and **everyone working with the subjects or subjects' data** were unaware of the study assignment. For how many patients did a blind need to be broken and under what circumstances? Was this comparable between groups?

As we will be evaluating the likely success of blinding, we are interested in anything that might help us determine that. However, we do not recommend that investigators attempt to "test the success of blinding." The results of this attempt may be misleading due to chance, and there is a strong possibility of confounding due to pre-trial hunches about efficacy as described by Sackett in a letter to the BMJ, "Why not test success of blinding?"[Sackett 04]. If you are interested, you can read more about this, including some scenarios, at this link on our website at www.delfini.org which will be accessible from the **Reader Resource** web page:

www.delfini.org/delfiniClick_PrimaryStudies.htm#blindingsuccess

4. Identify details about other care experiences

This information can be useful for external validity purposes for clinicians and others to consider what may help generate similar results in a patient population, etc. This information may also be important in assessing validity if there are differences between groups other than the intervention under investigation. The key area in which this can occur is in co-interventions. Using pharmaceutical agents as an example, we are interested in as much detail as possible to **help us understand if there was an imbalance of co-interventions** between the groups. In addition to knowing the percent of patients receiving which co-interventions, useful information includes dosing and duration comparisons. End-users want to know details about the study setting and care experiences in all study groups.

5. Intervention adherence

Report on how intervention adherence was assessed, and **report on adherence outcomes**. (Strangely, studies will frequently report on methods for assessment and then completely omit any information about results of those assessments.)

6. Exposure to the assigned intervention versus contamination or "migration to other study group"

7. Protocol violations

8. Potential impacts of time and change

For example, might the population under study have significantly changed during the course of the trial, such that later enrollees are very different than early enrollees? Might the time period of the study affect study results (e.g., studying an allergy medication, but not during allergy season)? Could test timing or a gap in testing result in misleading outcomes (e.g., in studies comparing one test to another, might discrepancies have arisen in test results if patients' status changed in between applying the two tests)?

9. Length of duration of treatment

10. Length of duration of study follow-up

11. Identify any other differences between the groups other than the intervention under investigation

Data Collection & Loss of Data

1. Report on what information was collected and how it was collected.

If using a **nonstandard instrument**, provide an explanation for your choice. For all instruments used, include a reference for the validation study.

2. Subject disposition

Provide the number of subjects assessed for eligibility, number excluded, number randomized by group, number discontinued and provide the reasons for discontinuation. Readers need to know how many subjects completed the study and how many subjects were included in the primary analysis. In reporting reasons for discontinuation, important categories include disease progression, consent withdrawal, patient request, adverse effects, administrative decision, noncompliance, loss to follow-up, protocol deviation, found to be ineligible, etc. Where relevant, we personally find it helpful to have "did not complete the study due to death" reported as a separate category and not include it in the totals for discontinuation.

It is especially helpful for end-users to have a **disposition chart** such as a CONSORT-style flowchart or flow diagram to display this information. Typing "consort flow chart" into an online search engine will bring up the CONSORT Group's template (http://www.consort-statement.org/consort-statement/flow-diagram0/) and choosing "Images" in Google will provide you with myriad examples. It is important to have the actual number of subjects, but it is greatly appreciated by assessors to include various calculations, such as the percent as well as the number in each category and the difference in percentages between groups by category. This is helpful to reviewers who would otherwise have to compute this by hand, a common omission which can be a source of extra work for reviewers (and yet another opportunity for frustration for customers).

This disposition information is not only of use to end-users, it might be more useful to you than you realize. Let's say you have large attrition in your study. Along with other considerations, comparability in reasons for discontinuation, especially if many categories are reported, may be suggestive that attrition bias was not present—again, setting aside smaller sample size issues. We have been able to use this information in several instances to perform analyses to "rescue" studies that were otherwise doomed for the chopping block because of high rates of attrition.

3. Report on missing information and its potential impact on results.

Missing data and patient attrition, which we will use to mean both missing subjects and subjects unable to complete study treatment, can create great consternation for reviewers. Ideally, study procedures are established to minimize missing data and patient attrition, and study staff work extremely hard to avoid these problems. However, at times it cannot be helped. When significant attrition occurs, it is important to understand that attrition does not necessarily equal "attrition bias," but may simply mean you now may have smaller sample size issues—but many customers do not understand this. When data are missing, including opportunities for data lost through attrition, authors can provide a great deal of help to reviewers by trying to **assess and communicate the likelihood of missing data to meaningfully impact study results**.

Assessing The Differences In The Outcomes In The Study Groups

1. Statistical methods used including disclosing the level set for significance

2. Assumptions for modeling

3. Population analysis methods

For superiority studies reporting dichotomous efficacy outcomes, we want to see an **intention–to–treat analysis**. Dichotomous or binary outcomes are those with two mutually exclusive categories resulting in "either this or that" such as "death" or "survival." We're happy to see the populations evaluated in other ways as well—such as completer analyses— but sophisticated reviewers, the CONSORT Statement authors and other major journal editors favor ITT analysis as being the primary analysis in these kinds of studies.

If performing an **intention-to-treat analysis**, be aware that the first thing that we are looking for is whether or not all subjects were analyzed in the groups to which they were randomized. Answering this directly is valued. The second thing that we are evaluating is how the investigators have imputed data for missing values. What we are seeking to understand is the effect of the authors' imputation methods on the results. We need enough detail and clarity in the published study to redo this assessment if we prefer a different method. If this information is not clearly available to us, and if we have concerns about the data imputation, there is a high risk of a study being rejected.

If performing a **time-to-event analysis**, be aware that the first thing we are looking for are the **censoring rules**. We are seeking to understand the effect of censoring on the results. Again, we need enough clarity reported to redo this assessment if we disagree with the censoring choices. If this information is not clearly available to us, and if we have concerns about the censoring, this too can result in a high risk of a study being rejected.

4. Results

For results reporting, when possible, we want to see reporting at the level of detail which would allow us to compute our own statistics, if we wish. In short, **we need the number of patients experiencing an outcome by study group as compared to those who did not**.

We want results reported in **absolute measures**.

We want to see **denominators** reported. It is surprisingly often that a percentage is reported, but we have to ask "percent of what?" When those who are sophisticated in evaluating medical evidence do not get this information, they will tend to supply it for you by taking the most conservative approach—meaning the outcome least favorable to your product. For example, if we see a statement that 12% of patients benefited, but it is not clear to us 12% of what group, we may choose to interpret this most conservatively as being 12% of those randomized instead of 12% of completers which might actually be what you meant. This could have a very meaningful effect on outcomes if, in fact, the denominator was based on completers and the differential between those randomized and those completing the study is large.

We think that sometimes analyzing the data in different ways can help mitigate uncertainty. Therefore, at times, we and many others value **sensitivity analyses** (i.e., "what if scenarios" that test the durability of statistical significance using various population analyses, data imputation methods, different statistical tests, etc). One example would be to provide results of both an intention-to-treat analysis compared to a completer analysis to see if results were similar. Sensitivity analyses sometimes utilize subgroups for data testing. Caution must be applied here, however, to make sure definitions and intentions are clear because *utilizing* subgroups for sensitivity analysis is not the same as doing subgroup analysis. The point of sensitivity analyses are to make sure the data stand up even in altered circumstances whereas subgroup analyses, *per se*, are attempts to isolate outcome differences in specialized groups. Caution must be applied because increasing the number of analyses also increases the likelihood of results being due to chance. Any *post hoc* analyses should be carefully labeled as such because these can only be considered hypothesis-generating and exploratory.

For **safety**, only patients who experienced an exposure should be evaluated, and they should be evaluated **not** as randomized, but as exposed.

We want to see **p-values** and **confidence intervals**. Reporting both is greatly appreciated by end-users who are frequently in the position of having to calculate the confidence intervals themselves.

If **composite endpoints** are used, we want to see the results for the individual outcomes that make up the composite.

An important bias consideration is **selective reporting**. Be sure to report results for *all* outcomes chosen as primary or secondary outcomes.

There are certain things that we have tried to point out that all reviewers are likely to pay attention to regardless of their competence in critical appraisal—and anything that sounds overstated or out of place or raises other red flags is likely to be jumped on by many reviewers. If your science quality is high, the last thing you want to do is jeopardize impressions and create a situation where your good work is looked upon with a jaded eye. When the study quality is good and the results are meaningful, the data should speak for themselves.

Non-Inferiority and Equivalence Designs

For readers who would like basic information about non-inferiority and equivalence trials, we have provided a 1-page summary of important considerations which is available at—

www.delfini.org/Delfini_Pearls_Basics_Comparative_Study_Design.pdf.

Non-inferiority trials aim to demonstrate that a new drug is not worse than the comparator by more than a small pre-specified amount, referred to as the non-inferiority margin or "delta." Readers need the **rationale and the basis for how delta was determined**.

Authors of non-inferiority and equivalence trials should always provide a **reference to the referent (comparison) study** and report on any information that supports the validity and clinical usefulness of the referent study. In addition to the validity and clinical usefulness of the referent study, we are also concerned about whether or not the **study of the new agent is sufficiently *similar* to the referent study**. We review key details such as population, dosing, duration, co-interventions, adherence, etc. Are the outcome measures the same in the studies?

We are also concerned about the potential impact of time which, among other considerations, may have affected efficacy for even the referent agent—such as changes in resistance patterns to antibiotics or in patient behaviors such as dietary changes due to public health interventions.

Reporting for Crossover Trials

Appraisers would like to see the following information—

Randomization: Were patients randomized to an intervention sequence? If yes, report on this. We are looking to see that this varies so that all patients are not receiving the same intervention at the same time.

Blinding: Report on whether crossover points were concealed and how they were concealed.

Timing: We are also interested in anything you can tell us about timing including pre-specification of reasonable cross-over points, carry-over effects of intervention or non-intervention elements and disease issues (e.g., considering issues relating to curative potential, disease fluctuations, rebound, seasonal effect, etc.).

Protocol Compliance

Documentation of key trial elements (e.g., randomization, concealment of allocation, etc.) provides transparency and additional information for critical appraisers. The CONSORT Group now requests investigators to include information about the location of the written protocol so that all stakeholders can compare the published study to the protocol or obtain additional study information not reported in the trial.

However, we need **confirmation of what actually happened for key study elements**. Frequent unexplained discrepancies between protocols and published trials have been observed for details of randomization, blinding and statistical analyses [Chan 08, Pildal 05]. Therefore, we prefer to see statements about what was actually done directly in the published study or in a post-study resource that is readily accessible (e.g., how concealment of allocation was actually achieved as compared to what was planned in the protocol). Appraisers need information about major changes to the protocol or discrepancies between the protocol and the published study, (e.g., unplanned changes to eligibility criteria, interventions, examinations, data collection, methods of analysis, significance level and study outcomes including planned subgroup analyses).

The bottom line is that protocols are useful to appraisers because they frequently provide important details not presented in the published study—but more sophisticated reviewers will be cautious about accepting information in the protocol unless it is substantiated in the published manuscript or such resource such as a web appendix of the study.

Protocol violations and, at times, protocol changes may affect study results by changing important study elements with resulting bias or unbalancing of the populations or interventions. Readers frequently want to see what protocol violations have occurred (e.g., non-compliance, withdrawal from the trial, receiving the wrong intervention, etc.). The CONSORT Statement recommends that the nature of all protocol deviations and the exact reasons for excluding any participants after randomization always be available to readers.

Diagnostic Testing

Because of the complexity of this area, in this section we shift styles slightly to elaborate more on the topic generally as well as discuss some challenging issues. We will describe what critical appraisers look for and let you extrapolate from that for ideals for reporting.

The goal of diagnostic testing is to determine whether a given condition is present or absent in a patient. New diagnostic tests should be evaluated to determine if they lead to the identification of individuals who could potentially benefit from other interventions. In most cases, new tests are compared to a gold standard or some other reasonable comparator. A gold standard is a test that is assumed to be accurate in diagnosing the condition of interest. Unfortunately, gold standard tests are frequently invasive (e.g., a biopsy), and clinicians will often accept decreased accuracy in a test if the test provides other advantages (e.g., if the test is low cost, non-invasive or results are quickly available). Ideally, the new test finds the same abnormality, and within the same time period, as other available options.

Critical appraisal of a diagnostic test includes evaluating the test for accuracy, predictive value of the test and whether improved clinical outcomes result from the application of the test with benefits outweighing any harms. New tests should be evaluated for accuracy by applying the tests to patients who are known to have the condition and subjects who are known *not* to have the condition. The results of this testing can be summarized in a table called a 2-by-2 table, so called because the table cells display "test results" as positive or negative and "clinical status" as condition present or condition absent. Measures of test function such as sensitivity (ability to identify true positives), specificity (ability to identify false negatives) and predictive values are then calculated from the 2-by-2 table using simple calculations.

Think of this like a general internet search on your favorite topic. A search that is sensitive casts a very wide net to try and make sure you miss nothing which may be relevant (true positives). This search is very inclusive. Literally think of a fishing net. Your search terms are very general. You capture all kinds of things, but you have decreased the chance of missing things you wanted. You just have a lot of information to look through to isolate those things. Test sensitivity is like this. A test with a high sensitivity means you have likely found a large number of people that are truly positive for the test. But that also may bring with it the risk that you have included in your "net" a large number of people who are false positives.

A search that is specific is narrow. This search is structured to weed out things that are not relevant to your needs (false positives). Thus, specificity is a hunt for very specific items—think of a computer search, using quote marks, to make the search very specific in which you will *only* capture—not broadly capture—matched entries. This narrowness might increase the number of hits you get that are relevant, but you might miss a lot of other information that is relevant too.

Key questions regarding diagnostic tests asked by critical appraisers include the following:

- Are the measures of test function (i.e., sensitivity, specificity, positive and negative predictive value) acceptable? Frequently there is a clinical need to choose a less accurate method due to cost or risk (e.g., chest x-ray versus lung biopsy). It should be emphasized that these measures of test function apply only to the studied population and are likely to differ for different populations.

- Was the test blindly evaluated by applying it to subjects known to have and not have the condition?

- Was the test and the gold standard applied to all persons studied?

- Does testing lead to improved outcomes or better value?

Anything that helps critical appraisers answer these questions should be reported in the published study.

We have already discussed the issue of intermediate outcome measures. One of the biggest issues in diagnostic testing is also the use of intermediate (aka surrogate or proxy) outcome measures which raises the possibility that the test may not truly result in clinical benefit. For example, premature heartbeats after a heart attack indicate a higher risk for cardiac death. But does identifying premature beats through diagnostic testing, followed by treatment with drugs to suppress the premature beats, decrease mortality? In order to know if the diagnostic test is clinically useful, RCTs are required to know that those subjects diagnosed by using the diagnostic test have better outcomes than a comparison group that did not receive the diagnostic test.

In summary, critical appraisal of studies of diagnostic tests involves both evaluating observational studies designed to establish accuracy and predictive value of the tests and RCTs which are required (with rare exception) to demonstrate net benefits over existing tests for people exposed to the new test. Reporting should attend to addressing answers needed by critical appraisers.

Screening

Because of the complexity of this area, in this section we also shift styles slightly— as we did in **Diagnostic Testing**— to elaborate more on the topic generally as well as discuss some challenging issues. We will describe what critical appraisers look for and let you extrapolate from that for ideals for reporting.

Screening is a type of therapeutic intervention that embodies elements of both diagnosis and treatment. As is the case with diagnostic testing, the evaluation of a screening test involves comparing the new (index) test with the gold standard or some other reasonable comparator.

The key issue in critically appraising studies of screening tests is whether early diagnosis and treatment through screening is more effective (i.e., achieves better outcomes) than waiting for symptoms or signs before testing. Screening tests can falsely appear to be beneficial when they are not. Frequently, improved outcomes reported from screening test studies can be explained by lead time bias, length bias (also referred to as length time bias), overdiagnosis bias or volunteer bias which may create major distortions in study results.

From our online glossary at www.delfini.org—

- Lead time bias: A bias resulting from a disease found through screening as compared to when it might otherwise have been detected. This kind of bias can result in a treatment seeming to be very effective if the lead time is long (e.g., "increased" survival time).

- Length bias: A bias that can occur when certain characteristics or conditions under study differ in the speed of progression. This kind of bias can result in findings favoring screening. An example is tumors. Faster-growing tumors causing symptoms will be more likely to be found outside of screening. Slower-growing, asymptomatic tumors will have a longer duration and be less likely to be found outside of screening. Thus, screening will identify more slower-growing asymptomatic tumors which could then result in a conclusion that screening helps prevent mortality.

- Example of bias affecting outcomes in a study of a cancer screening test: a test for cancer detects slower growing tumors (i.e., fast growing tumors are missed because patients with fast-growing tumors are diagnosed and die between screening intervals and are not captured by the screening test) resulting in overestimation of survival time from early diagnosis. Or worse, the test detects cancer at an asymptomatic stage in patients who would not have ever become symptomatic or harmed by the cancer.

- Overdiagnosis Bias: A finding of a disease at an asymptomatic stage in a patient who would not have become symptomatic or harmed by the disease.

- Volunteers have been shown to have better outcomes than those who don't (i.e., those who are recruited through active requests to participate), possibly due to the healthy user effect. In other words, patients who volunteer for screening may be "different" (healthier) from the larger population and may have a better prognosis.

Key questions regarding screening tests asked by critical appraisers include the key issues of diagnostic studies (reliability, precision and predictive value of the tests), but also questions about the benefits and harms of early diagnosis and treatment before symptoms are present versus later diagnosis and treatment after symptoms or signs of disease appear. The optimal method for determining the value of a screening test is to evaluate important outcomes from well-designed and conducted RCTs. Outcomes in the screened group are then compared with outcomes in the unscreened group.

Reporting should attend to addressing answers to these issues needed by critical appraisers.

APPENDIX D: DETAILS FOR "PREPARE TO CONNECT OVER THE EVIDENCE ~ Know the Customer to Interact with the Customer"

Apply skills for enhancing connecting over the evidence in your interactions with your specific customer in mind. This includes being able to assess your customer's climate for medical decision-making and their evidentiary knowledge and approach both organizationally and individually within the organization. This also includes being prepared to bridge gaps in evidentiary knowledge and skills. Have effective methods for addressing customers' questions.

In this section, we provide you with questions to pose and give you detailed information. Following these questions in this detailed section, we repeat each question along with key points in a **Recap & Short Summary**.

Prepare to Assess an Organization's and/or an Individual's Evidence-sophistication: Sample Questions

1. How do they identify studies for review?

Obtaining relevant studies for review requires conducting a systematic search utilizing the National Library of Medicine (NLM), at a minimum. Observational studies are highly prone to bias and should not be used as proof of cause-and-effect for the efficacy of an intervention, unless the results are "all-or-none results." As mentioned previously, "all-or-none results" is the term that is used when highly dramatic differences in outcomes between groups are observed. For example, before the intervention, everyone died and after application of the intervention, almost no one died. When all-or-none results occur in observational studies, they are generally considered reliable. But only well-done experiments with good study performance outcomes are considered truly reliable to establish cause and effect. If observational studies are used to evaluate the efficacy of your product, it is possible that this could result in a beneficial intervention looking ineffective due to the high potential for bias.

Observational studies may be useful in assessing safety. However, safety too is a cause-and-effect question. Therefore, the use of observational studies to answer safety questions should generally be approached with care, applying cautious wording and cautious conclusion-drawing.

2. How do they conduct a review?

In part 1 of this book, we have already detailed much about this question already in our discussion of an organizational approach (i.e., criteria for evaluation, formats for reporting, standards versus a contextual approach, review process, etc.). If the organization does not have a formal approach for conducting reviews and doing critical appraisals, it still may prove fruitful to pose this question to individual staffers because they might, independently, have a process they use themselves.

3. What weight do they put on blinding?

As we have already stated in **Appendix B**, in our opinion, successful blinding is one of the most important critical appraisal considerations. We consider it so important that we would expect that evidence-savvy groups would be very attuned to this study issue and weight it extremely highly, potentially dismissing outright unblinded studies.

Also, some customers believe that blinding only matters for subjective outcomes. As we have described in **Appendix B**, they are wrong.

Because of the very detailed discussion about blinding provided in **Appendix B**, we will not repeat that information here, but will detail points to review with customers both here and in the **Recap & Short Summary** that follows all of these questions:

> Do they understand and look for concealment of allocation of patients to their study groups? How do they value blinding? Do they give blinding different weight for subjective versus objective outcomes? Do they give blinding a pass if blinding is difficult to achieve due to the nature of the intervention or its application? Do they specifically look for a statement that assessors were blinded? And, do they attempt to evaluate the likely success of blinding?

4. How do they evaluate the use of co-interventions?

At its essence, medical research is about comparing differences in results between matched groups that are identically treated with one exception—and that exception is the object of study. Therefore, if co-interventions are the same in each of the study groups, this will have no effect on the difference between the results.

Evidence-savvy groups understand this. Reviewers who are not so sophisticated often misunderstand this and may believe that the results are confounded by any use of co-interventions—when the actual issue is whether or not the use of co-interventions has not been balanced between groups. Furthermore—

5. How do they evaluate placebo effect?

...we also see this same error in operation at times resulting in reviewers becoming confused about placebo effect, not recognizing that this effect will be equal between groups if the administration of the intervention is identical to placebo or to the sham procedure. Meaning, if a study is comparing the effects of an active medication to a placebo, the placebo effect is going to be operating in both groups *because* everyone is taking a pill, and any additive effect of the active agent or actual intervention will be revealed by the difference in outcomes between the groups.

6. How do they evaluate power?

This is kind of a trick question to pose because—as you may well know— *all* statistically significant outcomes *are* powered by definition. However, many customers do not understand that the definition of power is whether or not you had enough people to find a statistically significant difference if one exists. Many customers do not understand that the power calculation is only about trying to achieve a large enough study sample to discover a statistically significant difference if one exists and a small enough study sample to avoid waste, patient exposure, etc. Reviewers may incorrectly record a threat to validity if fewer people completed the study than estimated in the power calculation rather than understand that if statistical significance was reached, then the study *was* powered for that particular outcome.

What is not a trick question, however, is whether an outcome was sufficiently powered when findings are not statistically significant. A finding of "no statistically significant difference" between the groups—also referred to as "nonsignificance," "no difference" or a "negative finding"—may be misleading because there might have been a statistically significant difference discovered if the population studied had been larger.

So the correct answer is "statistically significant—or positive—findings" = sufficiently powered. "Negative findings" = two possible explanations. And when it comes to negative findings, a practical approach is to examine the confidence intervals to determine whether they include the possibility of what the reviewer, in his or her *judgment*, deems to be a meaningful clinical benefit to help address conclusivity or inconclusiveness of the outcomes. However, many of your customers do not know this.

Therefore, you need to be aware that misunderstandings about this area could cause some reviewers to falsely discount a study or study outcomes.

7. How do they approach attrition?

There are many published studies about the effect of various biases on research outcomes. Unfortunately, however, the research on the effects of attrition bias is inconclusive and, therefore, is of limited help. Because of this, none of us is operating on very solid ground when it comes to this research problem generally—although, sometimes the impact of attrition or its lack on study results can be assessed in individual situations. And, also unfortunately, frequently there is a lot of attrition in clinical trials.

Attrition bias is generally thought of as "loss of subjects to follow-up." And some reviewers stop right there. However, we believe the issue is a larger one and can pretty much be simplified by asking what data are missing. The important consideration is really about loss of data— regardless of whether it is due to loss of subjects or for other reasons, (e.g., data collection problems). Loss of subjects and loss of data can sometimes mean a loss of important information and/or it can sometimes mean a resulting imbalance between the groups that could affect study results. We will elaborate on both of these issues.

Some reviewers paint attrition with a broad brush and simply look at the amount of loss. They are not alone in this. For example, some journals have capped acceptable attrition at 20% (e.g., ACP Journal Club). Various reviewers have attempted to determine the risk of bias from varying percentages of loss [Dumville 06, Akl 12]. We believe that using a cap is likely to result in rejecting some otherwise reliable studies. Attrition is not the same as attrition bias. Attrition which does not cause bias merely results in a smaller sample, which may be a problem only if results are non-significant (i.e., the potential that too few people are now available for study to show a statistically significant difference if one exists) or if there is a greater risk of chance effects or outliers.

The real question is whether or not attrition bias is present and, if yes, has it meaningfully distorted results? For these reasons, we favor an approach that looks at the contextual elements of studies on a case-by-case basis. Considerations include how much information was lost, when it was lost, why it was lost and whether this loss is likely to have meaningfully affected results. At times, good study design, execution and study performance outcomes, such as successful blinding, can mitigate attrition bias even when attrition is large. Evaluating studies using these types of considerations to assess the likely impact of attrition bias is a more evidence-sophisticated approach.

Another variation in considering the effects of attrition involves whether there is differential loss between groups. There is general agreement that differential loss—meaning imbalance between the groups in the number of patients who drop out—generally points to some kind of issue with the intervention studied. Patients may drop out because of side effects from the intervention. Or it could be that patients on placebo drop out because they are not experiencing relief, whereas there are many fewer drop-outs in the intervention group because the intervention is working. Or it could be that lack of blinding has created a serious bias and so people on placebo are dropping out because they have discerned their study assignment and want an active treatment.

However, if the attrition numbers between groups are equal, there could still have resulted an important imbalance in prognostic variables between groups that could affect the study results. In general, if people in both study groups who complete the study continue to have similar characteristics, it may be reasonable to ignore the attrition at some risk of false negative results and greater risk of chance effects due to reduced sample size. In other words, if the completers' baseline characteristics ("prognostic variables") are similar to those subjects who were randomized, positive results might not be distorted from what we might see had there been no attrition. And so, a report of baseline characteristics of completers compared to those randomized can be useful as an indicator, but it cannot be counted on to prove that the completer groups are equivalent. It is important to point out that this way of looking at the baseline characteristics of completers is frequently not understood by critical appraisers and other study reviewers. Providing this information in the study and explaining its utility, may help avoid rejection by a reviewer if attrition is high.

8. How do they evaluate intention–to–treat (ITT) analyses?

The first question is whether or not the evaluator even knows what this is. As we described earlier, for dichotomous variables (meaning one of two choices, such as alive or dead), intention–to–treat, or ITT, analysis has been recommended by editors of major journals to be the primary analysis method for **efficacy** outcomes of **superiority trials**. ITT analysis requires that *all* patients are analyzed and that all patients are analyzed in the group to which they are randomized regardless of the actual intervention received and regardless of study completion or completeness of data. This requires the use of some reasonable method for assigning missing data points (also referred to as "data imputation").

Many of those reading studies are unfamiliar with intention–to–treat analysis. Of those who are familiar with this concept, many of them will accept an analysis that is referred to as ITT. However, sophisticated reviewers are generally aware that the term ITT may be used by authors of publications, but not actually followed. In fact, the term is frequently misused or a modified method may be employed instead [Kruse 02]. Sophisticated reviewers will ignore the use of the term and will compare the number randomized in each group to the number used for reported results, looking to see that these numbers are the same (and they should be the same people, but generally we have to assume this unless there is evidence to the contrary).

What many reviewers tend to forget to do is to evaluate *how* values for missing data were assigned. And this is extremely important because how the data are imputed can drastically affect the results.

In short, there are two main methods for imputing data: 1. methods which attempt to approximate the truth; and, 2. methods which establish a challenge for statistical significance.

Most authors employ methods which attempt to approximate the truth. Many statisticians favor using mixed-effects models. However, unfortunately the method typically used by manufacturers is last observation carried forward, abbreviated as LOCF. Most reviewers are not aware of the potential problems of LOCF, but more sophisticated reviewers note that this method is considered to be prone to bias and should not be used. (For readers who wish further information regarding LOCF, the following two references will be of value [Carpenter, O'Brien 05].)

However, in some situations when the study is of a progressive condition in which overall improvement could not be expected to happen without some kind of effective intervention, and depending upon certain study quality features, LOCF may be reasonable at least to determine the direction of the efficacy outcomes. Again, this depends upon meeting certain validity requirements as described here: www.delfini.org/delfiniClick_PrimaryStudies.htm#LOCFhelp.

Instead of attempting to approximate truth, some authors and some reviewers, including ourselves, employ a method which raises the bar for reaching statistical significance. If the outcome of interest survives that test (i.e., remains statistically significant), then it may be reasonable to conclude that the intervention works despite the missing data, provided that the study has passed a rigorous critical appraisal and is found to be valid.

Examples of times in which we will do our own reanalysis include when we are reviewing an otherwise valid study in which we did not agree with the imputation method used in an ITT analysis or for which censoring rules were not disclosed for a time-to-event, or TTE, analysis. In this latter instance, we cannot analyze the time to reach a specific outcome; however, we may be able to find an outcome that lends itself to an ITT analysis to help us confirm or find support for the direction of efficacy outcomes.

Some more sophisticated reviewers may do this kind of reanalysis work also; however, they may only apply a very tough test—such as "extreme-case analysis" which is a worst-case scenario method in which all missing patients in the intervention group are recalculated as "treatment failures" and all missing patients in the placebo group are recalculated as "treatment successes," for example. It's rare that outcomes for an intervention can continue to be statistically significant facing such a tough test, and less experienced reviewers or those with greater time constraints will be less likely to take the time to establish less difficult parameters that still put the intervention of interest under a reasonable challenge.

Also, many reviewers do not understand that generally ITT analysis should only be applied for questions of efficacy in superiority trials. ITT analysis is not appropriate for analyzing safety outcomes because it could mask important safety information. As previously stated, for safety, populations should be analyzed by treatment received, not treatment assigned. If a customer does not understand this, that could be injurious to your product's safety profile as well as obscuring important safety information. Imagine, for example, a head-to-head trial, in which a large number of patients with unfortunate safety outcomes were receiving a competitor intervention by mistake—but are analyzed in the group to which they were randomized (your product). Customers may need to be educated about the appropriate use of ITT analysis. ITT is not appropriate for non-inferiority and equivalence trials if the data imputation methods favor no difference between groups, which is generally the case. Most customers are unlikely to know this.

9. How do they evaluate time-to-event (TTE) analyses?

Time-to-event analyses are methods to evaluate the length of time to an outcome of interest such as time-to-cancer progression or time-to-pregnancy. Related terms include life table analysis and survival analysis which refer to the method regardless of whether survival is the outcome. Kaplan-Meier (KM) methodology is the most commonly used survival analysis in health care research.

Assessing the potential for bias in TTE analyses is important; however, many customers do not know this. One investigator with a special interest in this area reported that problems with TTE analysis may misrepresent outcomes by a relative 50% or higher [Lachin 00]. Time-to-event, or TTE, analysis, is a complex area, so only a few key points will be made here. But chief among them concerns censoring. Censoring can be defined as removing a patient's data from a TTE at a certain time in the trial. Investigators censor patients for multiple reasons. An important reason for censoring a patient's data at the study's end is if he or she has not experienced the event of interest by the end of the study. This is referred to as "right censoring" or "administrative censoring." Any other kind of censoring (also referred to as "non-administrative censoring") is subject to question as it may bias the study. At a minimum, censoring reduces the study size and can result in a greater likelihood of non-significant findings, which may be false due to a too small number of subjects in the analysis pool to show a difference.

The APPROVe trial is illustrative of what can go wrong with a problematic censoring rule. For one of their analyses, investigators decided that they would censor any patients who experienced a confirmed thrombotic event 14 days or more after ceasing study medication under the assumption that the harm could not be a result of the medication after this amount of time. This decision resulted in a radically different point at which the divergence of the curves became statistically significant as compared to not applying this censoring rule.

Such a rule should never have been applied. If it were true that the harm was not a result of study medication, that information would have been revealed through a comparison between the two groups. Luckily, this biased censoring rule was discovered by a reader who published a re-analysis after putting the censored patients back into the curve [Mundell 06].

All but the most evidence-sophisticated reviewers, with rare exception, have only a vague notion of how to evaluate a time-to-event analysis. Reviewers who are not looking very closely at the report of subjects evaluated at varying time intervals are likely to only look at the spread between the curves. Reviewers who are more analytical or data-sensitive will be alert to the decreasing number of subjects and will often throw up their hands in frustration and cry, "Where did the patients go???" Sophisticated reviewers will understand that censoring has taken place. They will look to find censoring rules to evaluate. Unfortunately, censoring rules are rarely reported. **This is a big problem, and this is one of our biggest and most frequent reasons for determining that the reported study results are** uncertain or unreliable. **Critical appraisers need to know information about the number of censored patients, the timing of censoring and reasons for censoring.** However, most customers are not aware of this.

We have rarely seen censoring rules reported in studies. At times we are able to obtain that information by reviewing the protocol or other supplementary information or by contacting the researchers. When we are unable to get this information, if a study is otherwise valid, we frequently try to confirm the direction of outcomes through other means such as doing our own intention-to-treat analysis, if possible, or assessing patterns in outcomes reported in different ways. Customers who are aware of the importance of censoring rules might take the time to contact the researcher. But we have rarely seen a customer take the step of doing their own reanalysis ITT-style for suggestive support for an outcome.

There is much more to address about potential for bias in TTE analysis; however, this is often as far as even the more sophisticated reviewers with sufficient time may go.

10. What is their process for evaluating clinical significance?

At the opening of this book, we discussed clinical usefulness—or meaningful clinical benefit—which concerns whether the reported results are large enough to benefit patients in clinically meaningful ways. The clinically meaningful outcomes are 1) morbidity; 2) mortality; 3) symptom relief; 4) mental, physical and emotional functioning; and, 5) health-related quality of life. Any other topic is an intermediate marker and requires a causal "proof of evidence" chain. So a key question is whether or not a reviewer understands this or not. (Some reviewers may use slightly different terms or have a few subsets, but their list should generally fit into the items above.)

The other key question concerns how they evaluate the clinical meaningfulness of the size of the results. This is a judgment which will vary among individuals and may depend upon many factors. Imagine yourself as a physician (and if you are one, this should be easy!) When facing a patient for whom an agent may be prescribed to reduce mortality, you may have a very low threshold for what you would consider to be sufficient benefit size. Now imagine yourself as a quality improvement department director. You are responsible for major organizational initiatives. You can only do so many projects each year. You have a limited budget and your charge is to focus on an entire population. Whereas the physician might say that he or she is willing to offer the patient an agent that shows any improvement in reducing mortality, as the QI director, you may decide that you need to realize at least a 3% benefit to make it worthwhile to engage in the very expensive, time-consuming and diverting activity of trying to change clinician behavior and implement a major quality improvement program. In fact, many groups will simply gestalt what they consider to be sufficient benefit. And this is not unreasonable.

And as we've already pointed out, many physicians and clinical pharmacists do not understand the difference between absolute and relative measures. So a measure of their sophistication will include understanding these, as well as the common measures of outcomes. Because of the frequent use of relative measures, especially by industry and newspapers, less sophisticated reviewers have been conditioned to have an overinflated sense of typical sizes of outcomes. This is unfortunate because it then frequently makes absolute measures seem insignificant. Sophisticated reviewers understand that frequently meaningful improvements may actually come packaged in very small numbers. You will want to understand where your customer falls—dismissive of small numbers or not and under what circumstances (which, ideally, should be very contextual). Customers who think that there is a "one-size fits all NNT" are lacking in understanding.

11. How do they utilize confidence intervals?

We've talked about this some in our discussion above about power. Confidence intervals are important for end-users because they provide a range of possible results that are as statistically plausible as the result reported. However, not all reviewers are aware of this, and reviewers who are less evidence-sophisticated may not think about evaluating confidence intervals at all.

There are also general misunderstandings about limitations of confidence intervals (and p-values too)—but that is such a complex topic that we will just state that there is a summary of these issues on our website to which we will provide a link at the **Reader Resource** web page.

It is also important to be aware that some reviewers mistakenly believe that, when 95% confidence intervals between groups overlap, this means that there is a lack of significance at the 5% level. In most cases, when 95% confidence intervals for two sample percentages or means overlap, inferences cannot be made about the presence or absence of statistical significance at the 5% level. This error frequently occurs when the investigators in such cases do not calculate the confidence intervals for the **difference** between the groups [Austin 02]. We have seen customers reject studies due to this mistaken belief.

12. Do they have special considerations for handling secondary outcomes?

This is an encoded question for two questions. The first is whether they dismiss secondary outcomes entirely. The second is, "Will you consider utilizing statistically significant secondary outcomes if primary outcomes do not reach significance?" At the immediate sighting of non-significant primary outcomes, many reviewers consider themselves done with their review. There are others—including ourselves—who do not take this position. We believe it is more important to look at all outcomes studied in a valid trial and see if there are patterns.

This is not an area of sophistication or lack thereof. There is some controversy about the legitimacy of statistically significant secondary outcomes if primary outcomes do not reach significance. Both sides of this controversy have reasonable points, and so at this time there is no good resolution to this issue.

However, you will want to understand the viewpoint on this topic of any reviewer looking at your science, and it is very likely that a reviewer who rejects positive secondary outcomes in the face of non-significant primary outcomes is unaware that this is an area of controversy. And therefore, this may give you an opportunity for reconsideration of your science if your primary has not reached significance.

Those who reject secondary outcomes in this instance fall into two camps. The first group is composed of people (such as statisticians) who are aware that the number of outcomes evaluated increases the opportunity for chance findings. The second group, which is the majority on this side of the issue, have simply been taught to reject these secondary outcomes without being provided with much by way of reasoning or a foundation for doing so. Frequently, people in this latter group will be confused about power, the relatedness of which we will now explain.

Our take is to look at the contextual elements of the chosen outcomes. Let us don the hat of the researcher. In our imaginary study, we pick as our primary outcome "reduction in mortality." Let us also imagine that we chose as a secondary outcome "reduction in cardiovascular events," a composite outcome consisting of stroke, cardiovascular death and myocardial infarction. Now shifting our hat from being researchers to being reviewers—if we saw in an otherwise valid study that all our secondary outcomes were positive (i.e., statistically significant), but our primary was negative (i.e., not statistically significant), we would *not* be thinking that we had a bunch of positive secondary outcomes due to chance. Mortality is a rare event and so not achieving statistical significance for this primary outcome may well be the result of having too few people in our study or having a study of too short duration. Understanding this can help you work with reviewers who are more likely to reject your research without thinking this through. But again, not everyone agrees with us on this topic in its generality—however, we think that even the most sophisticated on the other side of this issue, such as statisticians, might shift their position depending upon the individual situation, such as in the example we have just given.

13. What is their approach to all-or-none results?

Again, "all-or-none results" is the term that is used when highly dramatic differences in outcomes between groups are observed. These may be found in experiments or in observations, but usually refer to dramatic results in observational studies. Evaluating all-or-none results can be tricky because, if studies are observational in design (highly prone to bias) or are low-quality experiments, bias could explain the results. However, it is generally agreed by evidence-sophisticated reviewers that all-or-none results may be sufficient to prove cause-and-effect. Many reviewers, however, are not aware of this. We have seen customers reject a biased RCT where the outcomes were so dramatic and explanation for the outcomes highly unlikely to be due to bias because of not understanding this area.

14. What are their considerations for evaluating non-inferiority and equivalence?

This important topic is complex and such studies are being done with increasing frequency. We will keep our remarks brief, but much more information is available on our website at www.delfini.org where you can download a 1-page summary of key considerations for these study types:

www.delfini.org/Delfini_Pearls_Basics_Comparative_Study_Design.pdf

Importantly, many of us are not particularly comfortable with these designs. They serve a number of needed purposes, but their reliability is often tough to evaluate. While it is a truism that bias tends to favor the intervention, anything that is conservative against an intervention pushes toward non-inferiority or equivalence. Another issue, among many, is that the potential validity of a non-inferiority or equivalence trial is predicated on prior studies using a superiority design. Most people are not aware of this. However, for those who are, doing an assessment that involves prior studies now complexifies one's review, which can increase opportunities for errors or uncertainty.

In any event, the wholly understandable reaction you are likely to get to this question from any reviewer is a groan. And many reviewers are going to have no idea how to really assess the validity of these studies. But if you have studies of these types, you very much want to know—

15. Do they accept claims of superiority in a non-inferiority or equivalence design?

...which, however, is easier and more direct to address. A large number of reviewers believe that it is neither fair nor appropriate to conclude claims of superiority in a non-inferiority design. But guess what? Not only do we disagree with them, but so do the FDA and the European version of the FDA, the European Medicines Agency (EMA), and CONSORT 06 also came out in favor of this stance. However, the inverse (accepting non-inferiority in a superiority trial which does not report statistically significant outcomes between groups) is generally considered inappropriate. We would generally agree with the EMA that it depends; however, because anything that is conservative against an intervention pushes toward non-inferiority or equivalence and because of the complexities of doing these studies, we ourselves, would be unlikely to accept such claims.

16. What is their approach to secondary studies such as systematic reviews and secondary sources such as clinical guidelines, compendia, comparative effectiveness research and health care economic studies?

In this book we have focused on primary studies (original research studies). Secondary studies (studies including more than one study) and secondary sources (derivative works which usually include evidence from medical research along with experts' opinions) are used by many payers, health care systems and other groups.

It is important to determine how your customers utilize secondary studies and sources. An evidence-sophisticated discussion will be likely to include an acknowledgment that many secondary studies and sources are flawed because they do not include evidence that has been critically appraised and found to be reliable and clinically useful. We and others have found this to be true of many secondary studies, such as systematic reviews and metaanalyses [Brok 08, Egger 03, Hennekens 12-09; Hennekens 04-09, Le Lorier 97]. This is also true of many clinical practice guidelines (which are secondary sources)—even from respected groups [Grilli 00].

Nevertheless, some groups accept conclusions and recommendations from clinical guidelines. Medicare, for example, uses "evidence-based guidelines" along with experts' opinions to inform decisions and recommendations. Many groups obtain clinical guidelines by searching the National Guideline Clearinghouse (NGC), a publicly funded clearinghouse for clinical practice guidelines. Many of these guidelines, if critically appraised, might be found to be invalid.

There are many other secondary sources used by payers and, not uncommonly, different sources reach different conclusions about the evidence and, therefore, their recommendations also vary. Examples of secondary sources used by payers include The Cochrane Collaboration, the National Institute for Clinical Excellence (NICE), DynaMed™, Database of Abstracts of Reviews of Effects (DARE), United States Preventive Services Taskforce (USPSTF), Agency for Healthcare Research and Quality (AHRQ) and Veterans Affairs/Department of Defense (VA/DOD), to name a few. Sophisticated payers use secondary studies and sources primarily as benchmarks to compare their findings to those reported by the benchmarks.

If customers rely on secondary studies and sources, it is frequently necessary to evaluate the evidence upon which the conclusions and recommendations are based to determine if the quality of the reported results and conclusions is acceptable. A question for customers is whether they critically appraise these sources and, if yes, how are they doing so? There are many tools available for evaluating secondary studies and sources [West 02], and we have evaluation checklists available at www.delfini.org.

Health care economic studies are secondary sources that are frequently employed to determine both the effectiveness and safety of interventions along with cost considerations. Unfortunately, these studies frequently do not employ an evidence-based approach for assessing effectiveness—rather, they build models accepting studies' reported results without critically appraising the studies [Jefferson 02, Stone 05]. As with all secondary sources, it is necessary to evaluate the evidence upon which the conclusions and recommendations of economic analyses are based to determine if the results and conclusions are acceptable. Frequently, however, customers do not do an adequate assessment of these studies.

17. What is their knowledge of the clinical disease state targeted by your product?

Staffers for medical decision-making committees—even if they are physicians—may not have a clinical background in the disease state your product is targeting, particularly if it is a specialty product or specialty area. As such, the import of your product or urgency for review from a patient perspective may be obscured. Using psoriasis as an example, a clinical pharmacist might think of this only as a skin disease and be unaware of the burden of disease and other clinical implications—or, in the case of rheumatoid arthritis, the importance of early aggressive treatment. You want to know if they understand special aspects of the disease important for treatment. Understanding their knowledge of your product's indication may provide an important opportunity for a little education that may go a long way in ensuring a fair review of your product and helping patients.

18. How do they evaluate safety?

We've discussed various problems with attempting to evaluate the safety of an intervention. When it comes to published studies, often safety will only be assessed within the context of RCTs reviewed for efficacy due to the extreme time commitment usually required to evaluate observations. But it will be useful for you to know how they are evaluating safety and may provide you with an opportunity to share some important information that may be otherwise overlooked.

19. How do they conduct reviews of studies of diagnostic tests and screening?

Because of the very complex nature of these studies, we refer you to our discussions of these two topics at the end of **Appendix C**.

Recap & Short Summary: Questions to Assess an Organization's or an Individual's Evidence-sophistication

1. **How do they identify studies for review?**
    Do they perform a systematic search including the NLM? Do they only utilize RCTs, with rare exception (i.e., "all-or-none results,") to answer questions of causality for efficacy?

2. **How do they conduct a review?**
    How do they frame a clinical question? Do they take a class effect approach? Do they perform critical appraisal? If yes, what are their criteria and what documents do they use to aid in their review and for reporting their findings? Do they apply standards? Are multiple people involved in reviews and what is their process? Do staff receive training in critical appraisal, and are they evaluated for critical appraisal skills by others who possess these skills?

3. **What weight do they put on blinding?**
    Do they understand and look for concealment of allocation of patients to their study groups? How do they value blinding? Do they give blinding different weight for subjective versus objective outcomes? Do

they give blinding a pass if blinding is difficult to achieve due to the nature of the intervention or its application? Do they specifically look for a statement that assessors were blinded? And, do they attempt to evaluate the likely success of blinding?

4. **How do they evaluate the use of co-interventions?**
Do they understand that, if co-interventions are the same in each of the study groups, this will have no effect on the difference between the results?

5. **How do they evaluate placebo effect?**
Do they understand that placebo effect is accounted for in the difference between groups provided that the interventions are similar (i.e., a pill versus a pill)?

6. **How do they evaluate power?**
Do they understand that any result that is statistically significant is, by definition, powered? Do they understand that a non-significant difference between groups does not necessarily mean there is no true difference between the groups?

7. **How do they approach attrition?**
Do they apply a percentage-approach to reject studies? Do they understand attrition does not necessarily equate with attrition bias (but may be subject to smaller sample size issues)? Do they only pay attention to differential loss? Do they understand that balanced loss in aggregate may still mean study groups have become unbalanced in prognostic variables? Do they believe there is utility in baseline comparisons of completers?

8. **How do they evaluate intention–to–treat analyses?**
Do they know what ITT analyses are and when they should and should not be used (i.e., yes for dichotomous efficacy outcomes of superiority trials; no for safety and generally no for equivalence or non-inferiority trials depending on the imputation method used)? Do they place a value on ITT analyses? Do they know the requirements for ITT analysis (i.e., subjects analyzed as randomized, with values included for all randomized patients)? Do they know what it means to impute data? Do they understand, in at least a general way, methods for imputing data? How do they evaluate these methods? Do they know how to perform an ITT analysis themselves? If yes, what is their approach?

9. **How do they evaluate time-to-event analyses?**
What do they look for and what is their approach? Do they understand censoring and its import? Do they evaluate censoring rules?

10. **What is their process for evaluating clinical significance?**
    What do they consider to be clinically relevant endpoints? How do they regard intermediate markers? Do they understand the difference between absolute and relative measures?

11. **How do they utilize confidence intervals?**
    The first question is actually *do* they utilize confidence intervals and do they understand what they mean? How do they use them? Do they ever compute them themselves? What are their beliefs about overlapping confidence intervals?

12. **Do they have special considerations for handling secondary outcomes?**
    Essentially this boils down to how they relate to secondary outcomes. Do they ignore secondary outcomes entirely? Do they reject positive secondary outcomes if the primary outcome has not achieved statistical significance? If not, how do they evaluate secondary outcomes? What are their understandings about secondary outcomes and chance?

13. **What is their approach to all-or-none results?**
    Do they know what this term means? If yes, do they have an approach to how they evaluate such results?

14. **What are their considerations for evaluating non-inferiority and equivalence?**
    Do they understand that considerations vary for evaluating these studies as compared to superiority designs? What are their considerations? Do they evaluate referent studies? Remember that if the referent study is flawed, the agent being studied may not be superior to placebo.

15. **Do they accept claims of superiority in a non-inferiority or equivalence design?**
    If they answer no to this question, do they understand that the FDA, the EMA and others are in agreement that it is appropriate to do so for valid studies? Do they understand that they should, in all likelihood, not accept claims of inferiority or equivalence in superiority designs?

16. **What is their approach to secondary studies such as systematic reviews and secondary sources such as clinical guidelines, compendia, comparative effectiveness research and health care economic studies?**
    Are they aware that many secondary sources, even from respected groups, are flawed often due to the inclusion of flawed studies or studies of uncertain reliability?

17. **What is their knowledge of the clinical disease state targeted by your product?**
Do they understand key clinical information of import about your product's indication? Assess this organizationally and for individuals reviewing your product. Are there key aspects of the condition or disease that you need to be communicating?

18. **How do they evaluate safety?**
What resources do they use to evaluate safety and how far do they go?

19. **How do they conduct reviews of studies of diagnostic tests and screening?**
Refer to **Appendix C**.

APPENDIX E: RISK OF BIAS DETAILS

The Cochrane Collaboration is a well-respected worldwide group of more than 31,000 volunteers that conduct systematic reviews of randomized controlled trials of health care interventions. Keep in mind that bias tends to inflate reported results, favoring the intervention under study. In their review of studies in which study procedures and other study elements were unclear, they found nearly twice the "reported benefit" compared to studies of higher quality. This suggests that studies of uncertain quality were as biased as the low quality studies [Hartling 09]:

Effect Size Comparisons in 163 Randomized Controlled Trials (RCTs): High Risk of Bias Trials versus Unclear Risk of Bias Trials versus Low Risk of Bias Trials

Group, Relative Effect Size (95% Confidence Interval)

High risk of bias, 0.52 (0.37 to 0.66)

Unclear risk of bias, 0.52 (0.39 to 0.64)

Low risk of bias, 0.23 (-0.16 to 0.62)

In case you need some help understanding these results, here's what they say. The studies are about various outcomes, and we don't need to know what these are because that is not necessarily relevant to understanding what these data are telling us. What is of interest to the researchers—and ourselves—is about "size of benefit" regardless of the interventions and outcomes studied.

Firstly, there is a large body of research indicating that bias tends to favor the intervention under study. We see that played out here where the effect size of the lower quality studies (i.e., studies at high risk of bias) is double that of the higher quality studies.

The key to addressing our scientist's challenge that we told you about in part 1 of the book is in the "unclear" category. The studies at **high risk of bias** and **unclear risk of bias** are reporting *nearly identical* results, and those results are statistically significant in favor of the studied intervention. The numbers in the parentheses are the confidence intervals, which show a similar spread of equally statistically plausible results for each of these two categories.

However, the studies at **low risk of bias** tell a different story. While they also favor the interventions under study, 1) the effect size is less than half of the high risk or unclear risk of bias studies; 2) they are not statistically significant; and, 3) the confidence intervals are much wider, representing greater uncertainty. So much uncertainty, in fact, that they might actually favor the comparator (i.e., the negative number)—which we do not see in the confidence intervals reported for the lower quality studies or those with greater uncertainty about study quality.

The fact that the effect sizes in studies at high risk of bias as well as those studies at unclear risk of bias are so similar is highly suggestive that studies lacking clarity in study design, execution and performance, in fact, are likely to be at high risk of bias. When presented with this information, our scientist colleague nodded in surprised agreement and expressed that he was now convinced that complete and clear reporting was more important than he had thought.

We spend much of our time reviewing other researchers' work on evaluating the effect of various biases on reported research outcomes. What we see time and time again is that bias tends to favor the intervention under study. The results presented above represent just one of many analyses that further support this.

In a classic example that showed the tendency of bias to favor the intervention, one researcher retrieved studies of mortality due to acute myocardial infarction, comparing them solely on the basis of two potential bias issues—randomization and concealment of allocation, which means that the way patients are assigned to their study group is blinded [Chalmers 83].

In the higher quality studies in which randomization and concealment of allocation were done, there was no reported difference in the outcomes between the control and the intervention groups. As the studies decreased in quality, the results increasingly favored the interventions—but in all likelihood, falsely. Studies without concealed allocation reported a 5% benefit favoring the interventions. As studies further decreased in quality, (i.e., the studies lacking both randomization and concealment of allocation), the results reported a 10% benefit favoring the intervention—which many of us would agree is a pretty big difference between the groups, especially when it comes to mortality. However, the likely explanation for these differences between the reported results in the intervention group and the comparison group is the difference in study quality due to bias.

Subsequent to this study, many other studies have reported similar findings—thus, it appears that bias in research studies tends to favor the intervention under study, frequently resulting in research outcomes that inflate beneficial outcomes, making interventions appear to be more efficacious than they actually are—and sometimes making interventions appear to be of benefit when, in fact, the opposite is true.

Evidence-savvy customers understand that bias can magnify treatment effect. Low quality clinical trials compared to high quality trials have been shown in some studies to overestimate benefit by up to a relative 30 to 50% or more for each individual bias identified. It appears that multiple study flaws may further increase the likelihood of misleading results. As the Cochrane Handbook points out, it is not possible to accurately predict how much over- or underestimation of the true intervention effect is caused by a particular flaw in a particular trial [Higgins Section 8.2.1.]. However, researchers who study the effects of various biases on results by comparing study results from trials with specific biases compared to similar studies without the biases have frequently been able to isolate relative percentages of distortion in the studies they have reviewed.

The following are estimates of the potential distortion on results resulting from different biases identified in studies. Keep in mind that these numbers are what we have found reported by various researchers—however, the effect of a distortion of results by bias could be much less, depending upon specific study circumstances, or a discovered bias might not even cause a distortion in results—but it also could be that a bias causes a larger distortion. So this is mainly just to make you aware that bias can have a meaningful impact on study results and is one of the reasons why we and others critically appraise studies.

- Inadequate generation of the randomization sequence—estimated range of distortion of results unclear to 75% [Juni 01, Kjaergard 01, Savovic 12, van Tulder 09]
- Inadequate concealment of allocation of subjects to their groups—estimated range of distortion of results unclear to 73% [Chalmers 83, Juni 01, Kjaergard 01, Moher 98, Savovic 12, Schulz 95]
- Inadequate double blinding—estimated range of distortion of results unclear to 72% [Juni 01, Kjaergard 01, Moher 98, Savovic 12, Schulz 95]
- Inadequate blinding of assessors—estimated range of distortion of results 35% to 69% [Juni 99, Poolman 07]
- Loss of data (attrition bias)—estimated range of distortion of results 2 to 38% [COTS 07, Nuesch 09, Tierney 04, van Tulder 09, Lachin 00]
- Completer analysis—estimated range of distortion of results 56% with 44% early withdrawal [Shih 02]

APPENDIX F: DELFINI SHORT CRITICAL APPRAISAL CHECKLIST— INTERVENTIONS FOR PREVENTION, SCREENING & THERAPY

Important: This tool is in "shorthand," requiring understanding of the individual critical appraisal concepts listed or alluded to. We have already described other resources that you may find to help you further understand the details of critical appraisal, if you so desire. However, this list provides you with a roundup of the essential core concepts.

We use this checklist in two ways. We use it to aid in our teaching health care professionals and others the core competencies of critical appraisal. We also use it in our critical appraisal work. After we conduct a review of a study, we review the checklist to ensure we haven't omitted a consideration.

This is downloadable from the **Reader Resource** web page and our website at www.delfini.org along with many other tools including a lengthier and more descriptive checklist that elaborates on these items and including tools for critically appraising secondary studies and secondary sources.

General: Note sponsorship, funding and affiliations, recognizing that any entity or person involved in research may have a bias.

Study Design Assessment	☐	Is the design appropriate to the research question? Is the research question useful?
	☐	For **efficacy**, use of **experimental study design** (meaning there was no choice made to determine intervention)
	☐	**Clinically significant area** for study (morbidity, mortality, symptom relief, functioning and health-related quality of life) and reasonable **definitions for clinical outcome such as response, treatment success or failure**
	☐	If **composite endpoints** used, reasonable combination used — and used for safety if used for efficacy
	☐	Ensure **prespecified** and **appropriate** 1) research questions, 2) populations to analyze, and 3) outcomes
Internal Validity Assessment: Can bias, confounding or chance explain the study results? See below		
Selection Bias	☐	Groups are **appropriate** for study, of appropriate size, **concurrent** and similar in **prognostic variables**
	☐	Methods for generating the group assignment sequence are truly **random,** sequencing avoids potential for anyone **affecting assignment** to a study arm and **randomization remains intact**
	☐	**Concealment of allocation** strategies are employed to prevent anyone affecting assignment to a study arm

Performance Bias	☐ **Double-blinding** methods employed (i.e., subject and all working with the subject or subject's data) and achieved
	☐ Reasonable **intervention** and reasonable **comparator** used (e.g., placebo)
	☐ **No bias or difference, except for what is under study, between groups during course of study** (e.g., intervention design and execution, care experiences, co-interventions, concomitant medication use, adherence, inappropriate exposure or migration, cross-over threats, protocol deviations, study duration, changes due to time etc.)
Data Collection/ Attrition Bias	☐ Evaluate bias in **measurement activities**
	☐ Might **attrition**, including missing data, discontinuations or loss to follow-up, have resulted in distorted outcomes?
Assessment Bias & Chance Assessment	☐ Assessors are **blinded**
	☐ Low likelihood of findings due to **chance, false positive and false negative outcomes**
	☐ **Non-significant findings** are reported, but the **confidence intervals include clinically meaningful differences**
	☐ **Intention-to-Treat Analysis (ITT)** performed for efficacy (**not safety**) (all people are analyzed as randomized + reasonable method for imputing missing values which puts the intervention through a challenging trial or reasonable sensitivity analysis) or missing values are very small.
	☐ If **time-to-event analysis** performed, appropriate, transparent and unbiased. Evaluate **censoring** rules.
	☐ **Analysis methods** are appropriate and use of **modeling** only with use of reasonable assumptions
	☐ No problems of **selective reporting or selective exclusion of outcomes**

Usefulness & Other Considerations

Meaningful Clinical Benefit	☐ Clinically significant **area** + sufficient benefit **size** = meaningful clinical benefit (consider efficacy vs effectiveness)
	☐ **Safety** (caution re: new interventions, caution re: non-significant findings)
External Validity	**How likely are research results to be realized in the real world considering population and circumstances for care?**
	☐ Review n, inclusions, exclusions, baseline characteristics and intervention methods — this is a **judgment call.**
Patient Perspective	☐ Consider benefits, harms, risks, costs, uncertainties, alternatives and satisfaction
Provider Perspective	☐ Satisfaction, acceptability (includes adherence issues, potential for abuse, dependency issues), likely appropriate application and actionability (e.g., FDA approval, affordability, external relevance, circumstances of care, able to apply, tools available)

☐ **Non-Inferiority & Equivalence Supplement:** Absence of the following problems: lack of sufficient evidence confirming efficacy of referent treatment; study not sufficiently similar to referent study; inappropriate Deltas; or significant biases or analysis methods which would tend to diminish an effect size (e.g., conservative application of ITT analysis, insufficient power, etc.)

☐ **Diagnostic Test Supplement:** New test requires better outcomes or value. Test is compared to gold standard or reasonable comparator and finds same abnormality and within time period that does not result in a change in diagnosis. Test is applied to all or random sample of subjects with and without disease. Assessors are blinded. There is minimal bias from indeterminate results. Measures of test function are useful.

☐ **Screening Supplement:** Early diagnosis and treatments determined to be effective will improve outcomes more than later diagnosis and treatment. Beneficial outcomes are not explained by bias (e.g., lead time, length, overdiagnosis or volunteer bias).

On our website, we also recommend additional resources for understanding these areas in greater detail including our book—

BASICS FOR EVALUATING MEDICAL RESEARCH STUDIES:
A Simplified Approach
And Why Your Patients Need You To Know This

Delfini Group Evidence-based Practice Series
Short How-to Guide Book

Available at—
http://www.delfinigrouppublishing.com/

IN CLOSING

We hope that this book will serve readers by providing useful information for those working in the drug and medical technology manufacturing industries to help them bridge gaps in understanding the evidence review processes used by customers, some common customer needs and some typical customer misunderstandings. We hope that this information will help improve medical information such as reporting of study information in published reports of trials and other research. We hope that we have helped to increase common ground between industry and customers to help foster important dialogues about evidence which we believe will improve care delivered to patients.

REFERENCES

AHRQ 09
http://www.ahrq.gov/about/annualconf09/abernethy.htm
Accessed 01/03/2014.

Akl EA, Briel M, You JJ, Sun X, Johnston BC, Busse JW, Mulla S, Lamontagne F, Bassler D, Vera C, Alshurafa M, Katsios CM, Zhou Q, Cukierman-Yaffe T, Gangji A, Mills EJ, Walter SD, Cook DJ, Schünemann HJ, Altman DG, Guyatt GH. Potential impact on estimated treatment effects of information lost to follow-up in randomised controlled trials (LOST-IT): systematic review. BMJ. 2012 May 18;344:e2809. doi: 10.1136/bmj.e2809. Review. PubMed PMID: 22611167.

Altman DG. The scandal of poor medical research. BMJ. 1994 Jan 29;308(6924):283-4. PubMed PMID: 8124111; PubMed Central PMCID: PMC2539276.

Atkins D, Chang S, Gartlehner G, Buckley DI, Whitlock EP, Berliner E, Matchar D. Assessing the Applicability of Studies When Comparing Medical Interventions. 2010 Dec 30. Methods Guide for Effectiveness and Comparative Effectiveness Reviews [Internet]. Rockville (MD): Agency for Health care Research and Quality (US); 2008. Available from http://www.ncbi.nlm.nih.gov/books/NBK53480/ PubMed PMID: 21433409.

Austin PC, Hux JE. A brief note on overlapping confidence intervals. J Vasc Surg. 2002 Jul;36(1):194-5. PubMed PMID: 12096281.

Bassler D et al. Stopping randomized trials early for benefit and estimation of treatment effects: systematic review and meta-regression analysis. JAMA. 2010 Mar 24;303(12):1180-7. PMID: 20332404

Bombardier C, Laine L, Reicin A, Shapiro D, Burgos-Vargas R, Davis B, Day R, Ferraz MB, Hawkey CJ, Hochberg MC, Kvien TK, Schnitzer TJ; VIGOR Study Group. Comparison of upper gastrointestinal toxicity of rofecoxib and naproxen in patients with rheumatoid arthritis. VIGOR Study Group. N Engl J Med. 2000 Nov 23;343(21):1520-8, 2 p following 1528. PubMed PMID: 11087881.

Brok J, Thorlund K, Gluud C, Wetterslev J. Trial sequential analysis reveals insufficient information size and potentially false positive results in many meta-analyses. J Clin Epidemiol. 2008 Aug;61(8):763-9. doi: 10.1016/j.jclinepi.2007.10.007. Epub 2008 Apr 14. PubMed PMID: 18411040.

Carpenter J.R, Kenward M.G. Missing data in randomized controlled trials—a practical guide http://www.hta.nhs.uk/nihrmethodology/reports/1589.pdf.

Chalmers TC, Celano P, Sacks HS, Smith H Jr. Bias in treatment assignment in controlled clinical trials. N Engl J Med. 1983 Dec 1;309(22):1358-61. PubMed PMID: 6633598.

Chan AW, Hróbjartsson A, Jørgensen KJ, Gøtzsche PC, Altman DG. Discrepancies in sample size calculations and data analyses reported in randomised trials: comparison of publications with protocols. BMJ. 2008 Dec 4;337:a2299. doi:10.1136/bmj.a2299. PubMed PMID: 19056791.

Cohen D. FDA official: "clinical trial system is broken". BMJ. 2013 Dec 5;347:f6980. doi: 10.1136/bmj.f6980. PubMed PMID: 24309077.

CONSORT Statement is accessible at http://www.consort-statement.org/ as of this writing 10/03/2013.

COTS: Canadian Orthopaedic Trauma Society. Nonoperative treatment compared with plate fixation of displaced midshaft clavicular fractures. A multicenter, randomized clinical trial. J Bone Joint Surg Am. 2007 Jan;89(1):1-10. PubMed PMID: 17200303.

Deeks JJ, Dinnes J, D'Amico R, Sowden AJ, Sakarovitch C, Song F, Petticrew M, Altman DG; International Stroke Trial Collaborative Group; European Carotid Surgery Trial Collaborative Group. Evaluating non-randomised intervention studies. Health Technol Assess. 2003;7(27):iii-x, 1-173. Review. PubMed PMID:14499048

Dumville JC, Torgerson DJ, Hewitt CE. Reporting attrition in randomized controlled trials. BMJ. 2006 Apr 22;332(7547):969-71. Review. PubMed PMID: 16627519; PubMed Central PMCID: PMC1444839.

Egger M, Juni P, Bartlett C, Holenstein F, Sterne J. How important are comprehensive literature searches and the assessment of trial quality in systematic reviews? Empirical study. Health Technol Assess. 2003;7(1):1-76. Review. PubMed PMID: 12583822

Eklind-Cervenka M, Benson L, Dahlström U, Edner M, Rosenqvist M, Lund LH. Association of candesartan vs losartan with all-cause mortality in patients with heart failure. JAMA. 2011 Jan 12;305(2):175-82. PubMed PMID: 21224459.

Field MJ, Lohr KN, eds. Guidelines for Clinical Practice: From Development to Use. Washington, DC: National Academies Press; 1992.

Freedman, David H. Lies, Damn Lies and Bad Medical Science. The Atlantic. November, 2010. www.theatlantic.com/magazine/archive/2010/11/lies-damned-lies-and-medical-science/8269/, accessed 11/07/2010.

Furberg CD, Psaty BM. Should evidence-based proof of drug efficacy be extrapolated to a "class of agents"? Circulation. 2003 Nov 25;108(21):2608-10. Review. PubMed PMID: 14638524.

Giannakakis IA, Haidich AB, Contopoulos-Ioannidis DG, Papanikolaou GN, Baltogianni MS, Ioannidis JP. Citation of randomized evidence in support of guidelines of therapeutic and preventive interventions. J Clin Epidemiol. 2002 Jun;55(6):545-55. PubMed PMID: 12063096.

Glasziou P. The EBM journal selection process: how to find the 1 in 400 valid and highly relevant new research articles. Evid Based Med. 2006 Aug;11(4):101. PubMed PMID: 17213115.

Gotzsche PC. Believability of relative risks and odds ratios in abstracts: cross sectional study. BMJ 2006;333;231-234; PMID: 16854948.

Grilli R, Magrini N, Penna A, Mura G, Liberati A. Practice guidelines developed by specialty societies: the need for a critical appraisal. Lancet. 2000 Jan 8;355(9198):103-6. PubMed PMID: 10675167.

Guyatt G, Rennie D, Meade M and Cook D. Users' Guides to the Medical Literature: A Manual for Evidence-Based Clinical Practice, Second Edition. New York: McGraw-Hill Professional, 2008. Print.

Guyatt GH, Briel M, Glasziou P, Bassler D, Montori VM. Problems of stopping trials early. BMJ. 2012 Jun 15;344:e3863. doi: 10.1136/bmj.e3863. PMID:22705814.

Hansson L et al. Effect of angiotensin-converting-enzyme inhibition compared with conventional therapy on cardiovascular morbidity and mortality in hypertension: the Captopril Prevention Project (CAPPP) randomised trial. Lancet. 1999 Feb 20;353(9153):611-6. PubMed PMID: 10030325.

Hartling L, Ospina M, Liang Y, Dryden DM, Hooton N, Krebs Seida J, Klassen TP. Risk of bias versus quality assessment of randomised controlled trials: cross sectional study. BMJ. 2009 Oct 19;339:b4012. doi: 10.1136/bmj.b4012. PubMed PMID: 19841007; PubMed Central PMCID: PMC2764034.

Hennekens CH, Demets D. The need for large-scale randomized evidence without undue emphasis on small trials, meta-analyses, or subgroup analyses. JAMA. 2009 Dec 2;302(21):2361-2. doi: 10.1001/jama.2009.1756. PubMed PMID: 19952322.

Hennekens CH, DeMets DL, Bairey Merz CN, Borzak SL, Borer JS. Doing more good than harm: need for a cease fire. Am J Med. 2009 Apr;122(4):315-6. doi: 10.1016/j.amjmed.2008.10.021. PubMed PMID: 19332222.

Higgins JPT, Green S (editors). Cochrane Handbook for Systematic Reviews of Interventions Version 5.1.0 [updated March 2011]. The Cochrane Collaboration, 2011. Available from www.cochrane-handbook.org. Section 8.2.1. Accessed 10/03/2013.

Hudson M, Humphries K, Tu JV, Behlouli H, Sheppard R, Pilote L. Angiotensin II receptor blockers for the treatment of heart failure: a class effect? Pharmacotherapy. 2007 Apr;27(4):526-34. PubMed PMID: 17381379.

Ioannidis JPA. Why Most Published Research Findings are False. PLoS Med 2005; 2(8):696 701. PMID: 16060722

Jefferson T, Demicheli V, Vale L. Quality of systematic reviews of economic evaluations in health care. JAMA. 2002 Jun 5;287(21):2809-12. PubMed PMID: 12038919.

Juni P, Altman DG, Egger M (2001) Systematic reviews in health care: assessing the quality of controlled clinical trials. BMJ 2001;323:42-6.PubMed PMID: 11440947

Juni P, Witschi A, Bloch R, Egger M. The hazards of scoring the quality of clinical trials for meta-analysis. JAMA. 1999 Sep 15;282(11):1054-60. PubMed PMID: 10493204.

Kjaergard LL, Villumsen J, Gluud C. Reported methodological quality and discrepancies between large and small randomized trials in metaanalyses. Ann Intern Med 2001;135:982–89. PMID 11730399

Kruse RL, Alper BS, Reust C, Stevermer JJ, Shannon S, Williams RH. Intention-to-treat analysis: who is in? Who is out? J Fam Pract. 2002 Nov;51(11):969-71. Review. Erratum in: J Fam Pract. 2002 Dec;51(12):1079.. PubMed PMID: 12485553.

Lachin JM (filed as Lachin JL). Statistical considerations in the intent-to-treat principle. Control Clin Trials. 2000 Oct;21(5):526. PubMed PMID: 11018568. Erratum: Refers to John M. Lachin: http://www.sciencedirect.com/science/article/pii/S0197245600000921

LeLorier J, Grégoire G, Benhaddad A, Lapierre J, Derderian F. Discrepancies between meta-analyses and subsequent large randomized, controlled trials. N Engl J Med. 1997 Aug 21;337(8):536-42. PubMed PMID: 9262498.

Marciniak TA. Memorandum of June 14, 2010 on cardiovascular events in RECORD (NDA 21-071/S-035): FDA briefing document, pages 16-151. http://www.fda.gov/AdvisoryCommittees/Calendar/ucm214612.htm. Accessed July 9, 2010.

McKibbon KA, Wilczynski NL, Haynes RB. What do evidence-based secondary journals tell us about the publication of clinically important articles in primary health care journals? BMC Med. 2004 Sep 6;2:33. PubMed PMID: 15350200

Moher D, Pham B, Jones A, Cook DJ, Jadad AR, Moher M, Tugwell P, Klassen TP. Does quality of reports of randomised trials affect estimates of intervention efficacy reported in meta-analyses? Lancet. 1998 Aug 22;352(9128):609-13. PubMed PMID: 9746022.

Mundell EJ and Gardner A. Journal Corrects Vioxx Article to Reflect Short-Term Heart Risk. 2006. http://news.healingwell.com/index.php?p=news1&id=533482. Accessed 5/31/2013.

Nissen SE, Wolski K. Effect of rosiglitazone on the risk of myocardial infarction and death from cardiovascular causes. N Engl J Med. 2007 Jun 14;356(24):2457-71. Epub 2007 May 21. Erratum in: N Engl J Med. 2007 Jul 5;357(1):100.. PubMed PMID: 17517853.

Nuesch E, Trelle S, Reichenbach S, Rutjes AW, Bürgi E, et al. (2009) The effects of excluding patients from the analysis in randomized controlled trials: meta-epidemiological study. BMJ 339:b3244. doi: 10.1136. PMID: 19736281

O'Brien PC, Zhang D, Bailey KR. Semi-parametric and non-parametric methods for clinical trials with incomplete data. Stat Med. 2005 Feb 15;24(3):341-58. Erratum in: Stat Med. 2005 Nov 15;24(21):3385. PMID: 15547952

Ong CK, Lirk P, Tan CH, Seymour RA. An evidence-based update on nonsteroidal anti-inflammatory drugs. Clin Med Res. 2007 Mar;5(1):19-34. Review. PubMed PMID: 17456832

Peto R. Failure of randomisation by "sealed" envelope. Lancet. 1999 Jul 3;354(9172):73. PubMed PMID: 10406390.

Pildal J, Chan AW, Hróbjartsson A, Forfang E, Altman DG, Gøtzsche PC. Comparison of descriptions of allocation concealment in trial protocols and the published reports: cohort study. BMJ. 2005 May 7;330(7499):1049. Epub 2005 Apr 7. Review. PubMed PMID: 15817527.

Pitkin RM, Branagan MA, Burmeister LF. Accuracy of data in abstracts of published research articles. JAMA. 1999 Mar 24-31;281(12):1110-1. PubMed PMID:10188662.

Poolman RW, Struijs PA, Krips R, Inger N. Sierevelt IN, et al. (2007) Reporting of outcomes in orthopaedic randomized trials: Does blinding of outcome assessors matter? J Bone Joint Surg Am. 89:550–558. PMID 17332104

Psaty BM, Prentice RL. Minimizing bias in randomized trials: the importance of blinding. JAMA. 2010 Aug 18;304(7):793-4. PubMed PMID: 20716744.

PubMed FAQ: http://www.ncbi.nlm.nih.gov/books/NBK3827/#pubmedhelp.FAQs Accessed 12/17/2014.

Sackett DL. Turning a blind eye: why we don't test for blindness at the end of our trials. BMJ. 2004 May 8;328(7448):1136. PubMed PMID: 15130997; PubMed Central PMCID: PMC406365.

Savovic J, Jones HE, Altman DG, et al. Influence of Reported Study Design Characteristics on Intervention Effect Estimates From Randomized, Controlled Trials. Ann Intern Med. 2012 Sep 4. doi: 10.7326/0003-4819-157-6-201209180-00537. [Epub ahead of print] PubMed PMID: 22945832.

Schulz KF, Chalmers I, Hayes RJ, Altman D. Empirical evidence of bias. Dimensions of methodological quality associated with estimates of treatment effects in controlled trials. JAMA 1995;273:408–12. PMID: 7823387

Shih W. Problems in dealing with missing data and informative censoring in clinical trials. Curr Control Trials Cardiovasc Med. 2002 Jan 8;3(1):4. PubMed PMID: 11985778; PubMed Central PMCID: PMC134476.

Smith, Richard. Medical research—still a scandal. 01/31/2014. http://blogs.bmj.com/bmj/2014/01/31/richard-smith-medical-research-still-a-scandal/

Stone PW, Braccia D, Larson E. Systematic review of economic analyses of health care-associated infections. Am J Infect Control. 2005 Nov;33(9):501-9. Review. PubMed PMID: 16260325.

Strite S, Stuart ME. "What is an Evidence-Based, Value-Based Health Care System? (Part 1)" The Physician Executive, Journal of Medical Management. Jan/Feb 2005; 50-54.

Svanstrom H, Pasternak B, Hviid A. Association of treatment with losartan vs candesartan and mortality among patients with heart failure. JAMA. 2012 Apr 11;307(14):1506-12. PubMed PMID: 22496265.

The Economist. Unreliable Research: Trouble at the Lab. October 19, 2013.
http://www.economist.com/news/briefing/21588057-scientists-think-science-self-correcting-
alarming-degree-it-not-trouble
Accessed 12/27/2013.

Tierney JF, Stewart LA. Investigating patient exclusion bias in meta-analysis. Int J Epidemiol. 2005
Feb;34(1):79-87. Epub 2004 Nov 23. PubMed PMID: 15561753.

van Tulder MW, Suttorp M, Morton S, et al. Empirical evidence of an association between internal
validity and effect size in randomized controlled trials of low-back pain. Spine (Phila Pa 1976). 2009 Jul
15;34(16):1685-92. PubMed PMID: 19770609.

West S, King V, Carey TS, et al. Systems to Rate the Strength of Scientific Evidence. Evidence Report/
Technology Assessment No. 47 (Prepared by the Research Triangle Institute- University of North
Carolina Evidence-based Practice Center under Contract No. 290–97–0011). AHRQ Publication No. 02–
E016. Rockville, MD: Agency for Healthcare Research and Quality; 2002. PMID:11979732

van Tulder MW, Suttorp M, Morton S, et al. Empirical evidence of an association between internal
validity and effect size in randomized controlled trials of low-back pain. Spine (Phila Pa 1976). 2009 Jul
15;34(16):1685-92. PubMed PMID: 19770609.

Made in the USA
Las Vegas, NV
02 December 2021

35848079R00098